LISTENING VISITS IN PERINATAL MENTAL HEALTH

Listening Visits in Perinatal Mental Health focuses on how women and families suffering from perinatal mental illness can be supported by a wide range of practitioners. Based on the skills of attentive listening, it is designed for use by health professionals and support workers concerned with maternal mental health and the mental health of the family.

This accessible guide:

- covers the process and progression of perinatal mental health;
- discusses the types of anxiety and depression that may occur during the perinatal period;
- examines the impact of maternal mental illness on the infant, father and family;
- explores available assessment tools, such as the Edinburgh Postnatal Depression Scale;
- presents the theories behind the efficacy of listening and counselling skills, as well as the evidence that recommends this type of therapy;
- gives suggestions of alternative therapeutic approaches and further resources to explore around perinatal mental health; and
- emphasises the importance of looking after yourself and making use of supervision and peer support.

With chapters focused on listening to mothers, fathers and infants and paying attention to cultural diversity, *Listening Visits in Perinatal Mental Health* builds on the knowledge that many professionals working with new mothers already have about perinatal mental health. It focuses on developing the skills needed to put this knowledge into practice and includes case examples and follow-up activities throughout.

Jane Hanley is an Honorary Senior Lecturer in Primary Care, Public and Mental Health at Swansea University, UK and the Past President of the International Marcé Society for Perinatal Mental Health. She is also a consultant perinatal mental health trainer for the Institute of Health Visiting and the director of an independent perinatal mental health training company.

Mark Williams is the Founder of Fathers Reaching Out, the first organisation to make awareness of and support fathers dealing with postnatal depression and their families. Mark went on to become Local Hero at Pride of Britain awards and 'Inspirational Father of the Year Awards'. Mark has given motivational lectures around the UK where he uses techniques including visualisation, affirmations, and positive metaphors to instil in his audience extraordinary self-belief and unrelenting confidence in their abilities. He has spoken on many television and radio stations about the impact of this illness on men.

LISTENING VISITS IN PERINATAL MENTAL HEALTH

A guide for health professionals and support workers

JANE HANLEY

With a contribution from Mark Williams

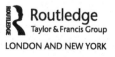

Routledge
Taylor & Francis Group

LONDON AND NEW YORK

First published 2015
by Routledge
4 Park Square, Milton Park, Abingdon, Oxon OX14 4RN

and by Routledge
605 Third Avenue, New York, NY 10017

Routledge is an imprint of the Taylor & Francis Group, an informa business

British Library Cataloguing-in-Publication Data
A catalogue record for this book is available from the British Library

Library of Congress Cataloging in Publication Data
Hanley, Jane, author.
  Listening visits in perinatal mental health: a guide for health
  professionals and support workers/written by Jane Hanley.
    p. cm.
  Includes bibliographical references and index.
  I. Title.
  [DNLM: 1. Depression, Postpartum – therapy. 2. Depression,
  Postpartum – psychology. 3. Empathy. 4. Family Relations.
  5. Postpartum Period – psychology. 6. Professional–Patient
  Relations. WQ 500]
  RG852
  618.7'6 – dc23
  2014047698

ISBN: 978-1-138-77491-9 (hbk)
ISBN: 978-1-138-77492-6 (pbk)
ISBN: 978-1-315-77422-0 (ebk)

Typeset in Sabon and Stone Sans
by Florence Production Ltd, Stoodleigh, Devon, UK

CONTENTS

ACKNOWLEDGEMENTS

The author would like to acknowledge the passion and works of both Sheelah Seeley and Cheryll Adams within the field of perinatal mental health, which inspired this book.

THE IMPORTANCE OF GOOD PERINATAL MENTAL HEALTH

'Perinatal mental health holds the key to unlock the mystery of mental health – we just have to locate it'

(Professor John Cox, conversation with author)

INTRODUCTION

Postnatal depression was a condition which concerned health professionals over ten years ago. It was recognised by society as a disabling and distressing problem which occurred to the mother following the birth of her baby. It was more severe than the baby blues and lasted longer. Some health visitors knew what to do, often general practitioners were consulted and sometimes psychiatrists and community psychiatric nurses became involved in the care of the mother. In some parts of the country there were mother and baby units which housed the mother with her infant, while the mother was being treated for severe depression or psychosis. Both were able to remain there until the mother was able to cope with her illness and was subsequently discharged. Care in the community was variable across the country, with no significant randomised control studies to support or negate the efficacy of the support networks. The services provided the best care they could.

Anecdotal reports suggested that many mothers, concerned about the severity the impact of their illness had, not only on them and ultimately their family, made a conscious decision not to have any more children. Had a mother made a similar decision following the advent of a physical illness, there would have been an outcry from society which would have ensured that science made a concerted effort to find a cure.

We have come a long way since then ... or have we? From a research point of view there have been radical and groundbreaking studies on the identification of depression as an illness. Other mental or psychiatric disorders have been identified, to include stress, generalised anxiety disorder, eating disorder, obsessive compulsive disorder, bipolar disorder, puerperal psychosis and schizophrenic disorders, which are known to have some effect on the unborn baby and the infant. There is currently more knowledge around the effect perinatal mental illness – the overarching term which describes conception to one year following the birth of the baby – has on infant and child development, the relationship with the father and the ultimate impact on society.

IMPORTANCE FOR THE FOETUS

Once revered, it is now disputed that pregnancy holds the same credibility, respect and esteem within society as it did in the past. Modern day living, coupled with the need for financial stability, has forced many mothers to work until late into the third trimester of pregnancy, and to resume working shortly following the birth of their infants, allowing little room for respite.

It is important to recognise the conditions that can be deleterious to a mother's mental health and have an awareness of the therapeutic and practical interventions designed to reduce stress and anxiety during her pregnancy. Good maternal mental health in the antenatal period will have a positive effect on the foetus and ultimately the infant, and should reduce any problems with the physical, cognitive, behavioural and emotional development which may have an effect on the child in later life and adulthood (Talge *et al.* 2007). To summarise, it is critically important to the foetus to maximise the mother's overall mental and physical health in pregnancy and after childbirth.

IMPORTANCE FOR THE MOTHER

Postnatal depression affects one in seven mothers (Wisner *et al.* 2012); this is an increase on the numbers given in the seminal work of Cox *et al.* (1987) over 25 years ago, which found that one in ten mothers were suffering from the illness. Overwhelming evidence during this time span has suggested that mothers suffering from depression in the antenatal period are more predisposed to have a depressive disorder in the postnatal period (Evans *et al.* 2001, Pawlby *et al.* 2008). The symptoms of depression however are no more common or severe after childbirth than during pregnancy, although they are usually more conspicuous after childbirth because there is considerable focus on the mother and baby.

The philosophical arguments about postnatal depression being regarded as a psychological state, as opposed to the continuum of mental well-being, remain unclear. Although it is recognised as being specifically linked to the advent of childbirth, often it is argued that it is difficult to distinguish the condition from the diagnostic measures for a normal depression, as reflected in the Fifth American Diagnostic and Statistical Manual of Mental Disorders (DSMV 2013). Nevertheless whatever the arguments, perinatal mental illness continues to be a challenge for mothers and their families (Goodman & Tyer-Viola 2010). There are numerous reasons why it is important to recognise and treat antenatal depression as studies have found several risk factors for antenatal depression which have been linked to poor outcomes for the infant, including prematurity and low birth weight (Shivakumar *et al.* 2010, Alderdice *et al.* 2012).

IMPORTANCE FOR THE FATHER

Men whose partners were depressed postnatally found the experience overwhelming, frustrating and stigmatising; overwhelming, because when faced with the plethora of the dispersive depressive symptoms, men often found they were unable to understand the insidious process of maternal depression which intruded into their life and that of their family (Conde *et al.* 2011, Gilligan *et al.* 2011). In one study Simmonds *et al.* (2014) found that almost a quarter of fathers experienced a mental health problem for the first time during their partner's pregnancy. The transition to fatherhood can be a time of risk for significant mental health problems. This is of interest, particularly if the father has a prior history of anxiety, which can be an indicator for antenatal depression.

IMPORTANCE FOR THE INFANT

It is not difficult to understand that if the mother's emotions are in a state of flux, she would find it difficult to bond with her infant. The word 'bond' has powerful connotations and presupposes that the mother has a strong maternal attachment to her baby; however this is not always the case. A mother who has experienced stress or depression during her pregnancy may often admit to neutral or even negative feelings. Whereas these may be common feelings, for some mothers, this may cause guilt, resulting in anguish, which only serves to exacerbate her feelings. This inability to express warmth and love might be unintentionally replaced with irritation and anger, not only towards herself but her infant. The necessary conditions for survival may be compromised, not physically, but emotionally. To secure positive development for the infant, it is important to provide the prerequisites of warmth, sustenance and love. All of this can be achieved by the mother who is mentally well, but can be negated by the mother who lacks those fundamental requirements in her own life. The long-term consequences have been evaluated and it has been found that there may be penalties for the older child as their development, cognitive functioning and behaviour may continue to be affected.

IMPORTANCE FOR SOCIETY

The World Health Organisation (1984) states that: '*Health is a state of complete physical, mental and social well-being and not merely the absence of disease or infirmity*'. The body of evidence currently presented clearly points to the impact on the infant's development which is determined by all of the attributes contained in that statement. This, in turn, will have a significant influence on the social determinants and the ultimate health of society.

There is increasing evidence that as the values and structure of society change and fragment, it loses the more traditional aspects of maternal and childcare. Therefore the need for good mental health should be a priority not only for local communities but for the whole of society. More importantly the recognition and management of deteriorating maternal mental health should be crucial to prevent serious consequences for the mother and her family.

Improving access to interventions either with psycho-pharmaceutical medication or interpersonal therapies, should be high on the public health agenda, and research into alleviating the causes of mental illness and efficacy of medication and treatments, a priority. If equal consideration were afforded to mental illness as it is to physical illness, a cure or at least a reduction in symptoms would be imminent. We owe it to future generations to ensure that there is a well managed perinatal mental health service, for if we are searching for a key to unlock the mysteries of mental illness then surely the place to start is at the beginning of life itself.

PERINATAL MENTAL HEALTH

Antenatal period

Women are at increased risk of mental illness during the perinatal period, and both perinatal mental illness and the treatment for these conditions may have long-term implications for their infants.

Anxiety

Anxiety is a common and understandable feature in perinatal mood disorders, but it is important to distinguish between what is a relatively mild anxiety or worry, and that which might indicate a more severe underlying mental health problem. Anxiety and stress is usually characterised by excessive worry, but it is difficult to control and causes significant distress. Common features are restlessness, irritability, constant tenseness and weariness. Concentration is problematic and the sleep pattern is often disturbed. The symptoms are usually experienced on more days than they are not.

Hyperemesis gravidarum (HG) may be a predictor of increased anxiety during pregnancy (Martin 2012). While an association between HG and mental illness seems likely, Kim (2009) found there is currently insufficient literature to support this link. However, studies have shown that women who suffer from severe HG are at increased risk of cognitive, behavioural and emotional problems during their pregnancy, and McCarthy et al. (2011) also found that these women had a higher rate of spontaneous premature birth, compared with women who did not suffer from HG. There is no doubt however that the thought of the transition from pregnancy to motherhood can be an uncertain time and for some mothers may heighten the risk factors of stress and anxiety (Emmanuel et al. 2009, Annagur 2013).

Other anxiety disorders with similar features include social phobias, post traumatic stress disorder, obsessive compulsive disorder, panic attacks, and eating disorders. Social phobia may have its origins in the teenage years. It is characterised by a marked and persistent fear in social or performance situations, in which there is exposure to unfamiliar people or possible scrutiny by others. For some mothers there may be a fear of humiliation or embarrassment when confronting strangers. The disorder itself can be a problem, but coupled with the thoughts of striving for perfection in motherhood, can lead to self-deprecation and in some cases, panic attacks.

Panic attacks consist of a range of anxiety-type symptoms with sudden onset and a limited duration, often lasting just a few minutes, but to the mother the time span is immeasurable. The cause of an attack is often unknown and may occur when the mother has felt anxious in a similar situation in the past. The symptoms can include palpitations, chest pain, choking sensation, 'butterflies' in the stomach, dizziness and feeling detached from reality, caused by hyperventilating. It is often frightening, and the difficulty in controlling the breathing exacerbates the feelings of vulnerability. It can be misinterpreted as an asthma or heart attack. Once identified it is easy to manage by reducing the pace of the breaths.

Symptoms of anxiety are also seen in mothers with obsessive compulsive disorder (OCD) which is characterised by recurrent intrusive thoughts, which can lead to repetitive behaviour. Attempts to resist the urge to carry out these behaviours can lead to severe anxiety (Zimbalidi *et al.* 2009, Abramowitz *et al.* 2010). Some of the more common behaviours include frequent hand washing and excessive cleaning. In the pregnant mother it might be obsessive thoughts about her unborn baby and often, in the case of the postnatal mother, it is the constant need to check the baby to ensure they are still breathing. It is believed it begins during the teenage years and can affect one in fifty people. Although not always easy to recognise, for the mother and her family the disruption to everyday life can be quite marked, as the obsessional and compulsive behaviour can prove exhausting.

Post traumatic stress disorder (PTSD) mirrors the symptoms of anxiety and is the collective term for a number of reactions which may happen to anyone who has experienced a severe traumatic or life threatening event. PTSD may be delayed for months or even years and is usually triggered by an incident that is reminiscent of the original distressing situation. This may be repeatedly experienced by flashbacks of the event and nightmares. There have been reports of mothers experiencing PTSD following a difficult labour or traumatic delivery and therefore it is important, as part of the therapeutic process, to encourage the mother to talk about her birthing experience (Garthus-Niegel *et al.* 2013).

Eating disorders are often caused by, or are a cause of, anxiety. One fifth of mothers suffering from an eating disorder also have a relative who also has the condition, though it is unclear whether it is hereditary, as a result of a dysfunctional relationship, sexual abuse or learned behaviour. It is possible for an eating disorder to co-exist with anxiety or depression.

The condition may be more apparent during the perinatal period as a result of the mother's personal desire or social pressure to return to and maintain her pre-pregnancy figure following the birth of her infant. It is of concern in both the ante- and postnatal period as both the mother's and her infant's nutrition may be compromised. Some women believe their body image is more important than the pregnancy, accepting the pregnancy, but not the inevitable weight gain. Some adolescent mothers, in particular, may be fixated with the populist culture that equates a lean body with beauty and success. However, while some make a conscious effort to maintain their weight while pregnant, others gain unnecessary pounds.

In some studies, it has been suggested that mothers whose weight increases exponentially during pregnancy were more likely to have been subjected to traumatic stress, but their equal despair at their weight gain made them prone to depressive symptoms (Molyneaux et al. 2014). The additional factors of decreased physical activity, fractured sleep patterns and fatigue may also be influential. Paradoxically this mindset makes it difficult to comply with fitness and diet regimes, while treatment with antidepressants may cause further weight gain (Atlantis & Baker 2008, Markowitz et al. 2008, Rogan et al. 2014). Rather than lose the extra weight post pregnancy, there is a tendency to gain excessive weight over the subsequent years, leading to further depressive symptoms.

The characteristic signs of anxiety and depression can be experienced in anorexia nervosa. It is often related to stressful life crises and may follow a traumatic life event. It is extreme dieting where minimal food is eaten, in some cases, resorting to a starvation diet. Excessive exercise is often undertaken in order to lose extra weight. It is a severe emotional disorder, which seldom appears before puberty and primarily affects three in one hundred adolescent girls, and an increasing number of boys. It rarely occurs in either men or women over the age of forty. Dominating and controlling parents have been identified as a factor for the disorder as by not eating, those affected are able to have some element of control, albeit as an act of passive revenge. The predominant psychological signs are a profound distortion of body image, because despite the extreme weight loss, there remains the desire to lose further weight.

Bulimia may be triggered by a traumatic experience, but equally may be used to manage distress. It is characterised by eating and inducing vomiting immediately afterwards or when it is convenient. Laxatives, emetics and, in extreme cases, enemas and diuretics are used to expel food. The mother who has been exposed to severe stress has been shown, in studies, to have low levels of dopamine and serotonin and higher levels of cortisol (Field et al. 2008). The process of denying or purging the body of necessary nutrients depletes the level of tryptophan necessary for the production of serotonin. In one study approximately one quarter of mothers reported their concerns over their weight and shape during pregnancy; binge eating was endorsed by 8.4 per cent, and 2.3 per cent of women engaged in regular compensatory behaviours for weight loss and to avoid weight gain (Easter et al. 2013).

An eating binge allows the temporary distraction from stress by focusing on the pleasure of taste and fulfilment of food. The act of purging regains control ensuring that any weight gain does not become an additional issue. The cycle of bingeing and purging usually becomes addictive, acting as a de-stressor but does not have the negative connotations of alcohol or drug misuse. Indicators are severe and often rapid and sustained weight loss, accompanied by the physical symptoms of poor circulation of the extremities, dry skin and hair.

There is still little research on the prevalence of eating disorders and patterns of perinatal mental health. Eating disorders are associated with an increased risk of adverse obstetric outcomes and may have long-term effects on child development. There are complex biological changes that include inflammation, HPA axis dysregulation, including the hormonal changes associated with pregnancy. It is probable that psychosocial problems around being overweight, the perception of body image perceptions, leading to poor self-esteem and poor control over dietary intake, make significant contributions to maternal well-being.

Eating disorders have an adverse effect on the growth of the infant, both physically and psychologically. While studies have found the infants of mothers with eating disorders were lower in weight, smaller in height, with a smaller head circumference, nearly half of clinically obese mothers have overweight babies and there is increasing evidence to show that there is the added risk of the infant gaining excessive weight during early childhood (Stein *et al.* 1999). There is undisputed evidence that perinatal stress and in particular chronic maternal stress may exert a significant influence on the foetus and the developmental outcomes (Talge *et al.* 2007).

Postnatal period

The description of depression in the postnatal period is often split into three sections, which include 'the blues', mild to moderate depression and severe postnatal depression.

The blues are now considered as a precursor to postnatal depression. Once regarded as a fleeting phenomenon, there is now evidence to suggest that the severity and duration of the blues is often indicative of possible postnatal depression (Henshaw *et al.* 2004). The mother is often teary and emotional for inexplicable reasons, and in the majority of cases this is temporary, but if her low mood is pervasive and persistent then it is worthy of further investigation to rule out any signs of a more severe depressive state.

PERINATAL DEPRESSION

The symptoms may be familiar in both the ante- and postnatal period but what makes it particularly significant in relation to other depressive symptoms is the addition of the foetus and infant. The fundamental signs of depression in the mother are the persistent and pervasive low mood resulting from a loss of pleasure or interest in her infant, her partner or life in general. Other symptoms may include psychomotor agitation or retardation, poor concentration, altered appetite and/or sleep deprivation. All of these emotions may have a detrimental effect on the mother but are exacerbated because it will undoubtedly affect the relationship with the father and the infant.

The mother may harbour suicidal thoughts and it is not uncommon for some mothers to consider taking their life should they endure the feelings of hopelessness and helplessness, resulting in feelings of inadequacy as a mother, lover and woman.

PATERNAL DEPRESSION

There is increasing evidence that fathers can also suffer from depression in the perinatal period. Maternal depression was identified as the strongest predictor of paternal depression (Goodman 2008, Schumacher *et al.* 2008). The rates of paternal depression have been found to range from 7–10.3 per cent and from 24 per cent to 50 per cent among men whose partners were experiencing postpartum depression (Goodman 2008, Bergstrom 2013). Paternal depression is associated with marital conflict and deteriorating disharmony within the partnership (Mao *et al.* 2011, Hanington *et al.* 2012). Postnatal parental depression increases the risk of adolescent depression, although the effect is mainly indirect through recurrent parental depression (Davé *et al.* 2010).

DRUGS/ALCOHOL

A cross-cutting theme is the co-morbid features of alcohol or substance misuse, either illicit or prescribed. Studies suggest that over 90 per cent of pregnant women take prescription or non-prescription drugs, illicit drugs or use the social drugs of tobacco and alcohol, at some time during their pregnancy. However, depressed parents are more likely to misuse drugs and alcohol in particular.

The overuse of the recreational drug cocaine increases the risk of adverse outcomes in the pregnancy, which may include separation of the placenta, retarded cerebral growth, poor development of organs, poor development of limbs and intra-uterine death.

High levels of consumption of alcohol, particularly binge drinking, may result in a reduction in infant birth weight and may cause a minority of infants to present with 'Foetal Alcohol Syndrome' whose features include a reduction in all parameters of growth, particularly the head circumference. This has consequences for neural development, central nervous dysfunction and the characteristic dysmorphic facial features.

PSYCHOSIS

Some mothers may experience a condition known as puerperal psychosis. There is still limited literature on why this occurs and for some mothers it is a single episode which does not reoccur following subsequent pregnancies. The first event usually occurs rapidly within days of the birth and is therefore a phenomenon seen, in the main, by midwives. Studies have shown it affects relatively few women, no more than one in five hundred pregnancies (Gentile 2010). The effects, however, are distressing for the family and disturbing for the mother. The behaviour of the mother may be disorganised and for her is distinctly abnormal.

As all of her senses may be affected there is a possibility she may see bizarre visions or experience auditory hallucinations which suggest a threat to her or her infant. Distortion of her sense of smell or taste may cause her to be secretive or suspicious as she believes in conspiracies to harm her or her infant. She may harbour feelings of paranoia or become obsessive in the hope of affording protection to both her and her infant. As the mother lacks insight she has the overwhelming need to react, which may compromise the safety of her infant and her own well-being. Some of the data suggest that it is probable that puerperal psychosis is an overt presentation of bipolar disorder (Sit *et al.* 2006, Doucet *et al.* 2009, Rusaka & Rancans 2014).

BIPOLAR DISORDER

Childbirth is a time of considerable risk for women with bipolar disorder. Around half of postnatal episodes occur following delivery and the most severe forms of postnatal mood disorder – puerperal or postnatal psychosis – occurs in one in five deliveries. This corresponds to a significant increase, compared with the general population, which has a rate of one in one thousand. The management of women with bipolar disorder is important in both pregnancy and childbirth.

Previously known as manic depression, bipolar disorder causes severe shifts in the mother's mood function. When it is at its most severe, bipolar disorder can cause episodes of extreme mania followed by dramatic and plummeting levels of mood. The signs of mania are the opposite of those experienced during a depressive phase. The mother's mood may be excessively euphoric, with rapid thought processes. The speech is verbose and often incoherent and her ideas are usually superficial and disjointed. She may suffer from the loss of inhibitions, delusions of grandeur, euphoric mood or irritability. Her concentration is affected which means she is unable to sustain tasks and is easily distracted.

Wisner *et al.* (2013) found that 22 per cent of women who had a major depression, had bipolar disorder, the majority of whom had not been diagnosed. Identifying the disorder depends on not only recognising the depressive phase but equally on the manic phase. Munk-Olsen *et al.* (2012) found that a psychiatric episode in the immediate postpartum period significantly predicted conversion to bipolar affective disorder during the follow-up period. Although there are many social and environmental factors which may predispose mothers to bipolar disorder, there is almost certainly a genetic factor (Green *et al.* 2013). Women with a family history (first degree relative) or personal history of bipolar disorder have a significantly higher risk of developing puerperal psychosis. The postnatal period poses the highest risk period for new episodes of mania in a woman's life.

The importance of managing bipolar disorder is recognised across the world and data presented in scientific research correspond with most of the studies. Studies in India found that the majority of mothers with bipolar disorder had some symptoms of depression culminating in low mood, suicidal ideation, pessimistic thoughts, impaired concentration, while some had the core symptoms of depression. These studies highlight the fact that depressive symptoms are common in women with postnatal onset mania and that in a small number, this may be severe (Chandra *et al.* 2006, Sharma *et al.* 2013, Ganjekar *et al.* 2014).

In America a study by Meltzer-Brody *et al.* (2014) found that approximately 18 per cent of the mothers admitted to hospital for bipolar disorder presented either with a history of or new onset bipolar disorder and/or postpartum psychosis. It was recognised that the mothers became critically ill, requiring specialised and targeted treatments which were sympathetic to both the mother's and her family's needs.

Women with bipolar disorder should be able to access preconception counselling, be monitored throughout their pregnancy and postnatal period and be treated when they have a postnatal episode both in the community and by admission to a mother and baby unit. However there is always the possibility that during a home visit they will express the need to be listened to.

SCHIZOPHRENIA

Schizophrenia translated from Greek means 'split' and 'mind'. This has been misinterpreted to mean that the person is in two minds and acts as separate people, but a more correct explanation is the differentials in the mother's cognitive and the affective functioning. It is estimated that over 1 per cent of the population has the illness. Schizophrenia was once believed to have been the result of a dysfunctional family; however there is little evidence to support this. Stress has been found to exacerbate the illness, and it is often precipitated by a life crisis. Some research has indicated that the biological response to stress is impaired as their cortisol response to stress is blunted (Gentile 2010).

Schizophrenia is characterised by marked disturbances in the mother's thought processes and perception of life. The prime symptom is bizarre behaviour, which is usually generated by a distortion of reality that is manifested in hallucinations and delusions. This may result in an insignificant association between what the mother is actually saying and the emotions she is expressing. Her fears may be articulated as anger and her joy as despair. This confusional state often results in the mother becoming preoccupied with her thoughts, unable to concentrate on her own reality, making her appear disinterested or indifferent towards her infant. These negative symptoms gradually erode her normal functioning, causing the mother to become more withdrawn and obscure. The complexities of the illness sometimes make diagnosis difficult, but it is probably the most serious and most debilitating of all mental disorders.

There is evidence to suggest that the use of cannabis is a risk factor for schizophrenia. Arendt *et al.* (2008) found that cannabis-induced psychotic disorders were diagnosed in just under half of the sample population. Frequent and extreme consumers of cannabis are significantly more likely to be diagnosed with schizophrenia than those who abstain.

MEDICATION

Some mothers report that they are reluctant to use pharmacological interventions, fearing the impact the medication may have on the foetus. Dennis and Dowswell (2013) acknowledge from their similar research that women are less likely to take medication for antenatal depression. Austin and Sullivan (2012) suggested that psychotropic drugs cross through the placenta, but what impact this has on the foetus has not been fully researched and currently shows mixed results.

Data about the rates and characteristics of antenatal psychotropic prescribing in the UK are however lacking, and the timely identification and management of women at increased risk of perinatal mental illness remains of critical importance (Petersen *et al.* 2011). More women are being prescribed antipsychotic and antidepressant drugs in pregnancy. Reports from various studies have indicated the safety of antipsychotic medication use in pregnancy for women who require these medications for their psychiatric stability (NICE 2007, Toh *et al.* 2013, Gentile 2010).

The use of medication during pregnancy is also the subject of a European drug project called EUROmediCAT which is designed to build a European system for reproductive safety evaluation. The objective is to identify systematically and comprehensively the possible adverse effects in pregnancy of drugs at the earliest possible stage. The study will monitor and evaluate European safety measures and will cover at least 3.7 million births from 1995 to 2010. This is essential for the study of rare outcomes – congenital anomalies and rare drug exposures. The EUROmediCAT surveillance system and the component national congenital anomaly registers aim to prevent a disaster on the scale of thalidomide happening again by detecting problems as early as possible (Charlton *et al.* 2014).

CONCLUSION

Ignoring the recognition, detection and management of perinatal mental illness can have enduring effects on the mother, her partner and family relationships as well as the mental health and social adjustment of the child. The worst case scenario is the possibility of an increased risk of the mother's mortality and morbidity. It has been suggested by theorists of functional analysis that poor perinatal mental health is a consequence of social deterioration rather than a purely physical reaction to the situation of motherhood. For many women societal factors may be an attempt to restrain and direct the rights of women, who may feel obliged to agree with modern day feminist thinking regarding their 'rights' to freedom, but also need to embrace their triple role of wife, mother and worker.

It is probable that women from a previous era would have felt the same pressures and stresses, had they shared the same lifestyle of today's women. However, women have redefined their role in society in past years and as a result there may be gains and losses which may inevitably affect childcare responsibilities and partnerships between mothers and fathers. There is a poor evidence base on the incidence of paternal depression and as the research emerges, it suggests that there is a profound lack of recognition and ultimately of the resources for fathers which need to be addressed.

REFERENCES

Abramowitz, J.S., Meltzer-Brody, S., Leserman, J., Killenberg, S., Rinaldi, K., Mahaffey, B.L. & Pedersen, C. (2010). Obsessional thoughts and compulsive behaviors in a sample of women with postpartum mood symptoms. *Archives of Women's Mental Health* 13:523–530

Alderdice, F., McNeil, J. & Lynn, F. (2012). A systematic review of systematic reviews of interventions to improve maternal mental health and well-being. *Midwifery* 29:389–399

American Psychiatric Association (2013). *Diagnostic and Statistical Manual of Mental Disorders* (5th edn). Arlington, VA: American Psychiatric Publishing

Annagur, B. (2013). Do psychiatric disorders continue during pregnancy in women with hyperemesis gravidarum: a prospective study. *General Hospital Psychiatry* 35:492–496

Arendt, M., Mortensen, P.B., Rosenberg, R., Pedersen, C.B. & Waltoft, B.L. (2008). Familial predisposition for psychiatric disorder: Comparison of subjects treated for cannabis-induced psychosis and schizophrenia. *Archives of General Psychiatry* 65:1269–1274

Atlantis, E. & Baker, M. (2008). Obesity effects on depression: systematic review of epidemiological studies. *International Journal of Obesity* 32:881–891

Austin, M.P. & Sullivan, E. (2012). The need to evaluate public health reforms: Australian perinatal mental health initiatives. *Australian and New Zealand Journal of Public Health* 36(3):208–211

Bergstrom, M. (2013). Depressive symptoms in new first-time fathers: Associations with age, sociodemographic characteristics, and antenatal psychological well-being. *Birth: Issues in Perinatal Care* 40(1):32–38

Chandra, P.S., Bhargavaraman, R.P., Raghunandan, V.N. & Shaligram, D. (2006). Delusions related to infant and their association with mother-infant interactions in postpartum psychotic disorders. *Archives of Women's Mental Health* 9(5):285–288

Charlton, R.A., Jordan, S., Pierini, A., Garne, E., Neville, A.J., Hansen, A.V., Gini, R., Thayer, D., Tingay, K., Puccini, A., Bos, H.J., Nybo Andersen, A.M., Sinclair, M., Dolk, H. & de Jong-van den Berg, L.T.W. (2014). SSRI use before, during and after pregnancy: a population-based study in 6 European regions.

BJOG: An International Journal of Obstetrics and Gynecology Article first published online: 28 October 2014. DOI: 10.1111/1471-0528.13143

Conde, A., Figueiredo, B. & Bifulco, A. (2011). Attachment style and psychological adjustment in couples. *Attachment & Human Development* 13(3): 271–291

Cox, J.L., Holden, J.M. & Sagovsky, R. (1987). Detection of postnatal depression. Development of the 10-item Edinburgh Postnatal Depression Scale. *British Journal of Psychiatry* 150:782–786

Davé, S., Petersen, I., Sherr, L. & Nazareth, I. (2010). Incidence of maternal and paternal depression in primary care: a cohort study using a primary care database. *Archives of Pediatrics & Adolescent Medicine* 164:1038–1044

Dennis, C.L. & Dowswell, T. (2013). Interventions (other than pharmacological, psychosocial or psychological) for treating antenatal depression (Review). *The Cochrane Collaboration. The Cochrane Library* 7

Doucet, S., Dennis, C., Letourneau, N. & Blackmore, E. (2009). Differentiation and clinical implications of postpartum depression and postpartum psychosis. *Journal of Obstetric Gynecologic and Neonatal Nursing* 38(3):269–279

Easter, A., Bye, A., Taborelli, E., Corfield, F., Schmidt, U., Treasure, J. & Micali, N. (2013). Recognising the symptoms: how common are eating disorders in pregnancy? *European Eating Disorder Review* 21(4):340–344

Emmanuel, N., Creedy, D., St John, W. & Brown, C. (2009). Maternal role development: the impact of maternal distress and social support following childbirth. *Midwifery* 27:265–272

Evans, J., Heron, J., Francomb, H., Oke, S. & Golding, J. (2001). Cohort study of Depressed Mood during Pregnancy and After Childbirth. *BMJ* 323(7307): 257–260

Field, T., Deeds, O., Diego, M., Hernandez-Reif, M., Gauler, A., Sullivan, S., Wilson, D. & Nearing, G. (2008). Benefits of Combining massage therapy with group interpersonal psychotherapy in prenatally depressed women. *Journal of Bodywork & Movement Therapies* 13:297–303

Ganjekar, S., Desai, G. & Chandra, P.S. (2014). A comparative study of psychopathology, symptom severity, and short-term outcome of postpartum and non postpartum mania. *Bipolar Disorder* 16(1):16–21

Garthus-Niegel, S., von Soest, T., Vollrat, M.E. & Eberhard-Gran, M. (2013). The impact of subjective birth experiences on post-traumatic stress symptoms: a longitudinal study. *Archives of Women's Mental Health* 16:1–10

Gentile, S. (2010). Antipsychotic therapy during early and late pregnancy. A systematic review. *Schizophrenia Bulletin* 36(3):518–544

Gilligan, P., Manby, M. & Pickburn, C. (2011). Fathers' involvement in children's services: Exploring local and national issues in 'Moorlandstown'. *British Journal of Social Work Advance Access*, published online 26 May

Goodman, J.H. (2008). Influences of maternal postpartum depression on fathers and on father-infant interaction. *Infant Mental Health Journal* 129(6):624–643

Goodman, J.H. & Tyer-Viola, L. (2010). Detection, treatment, and referral of perinatal depression and anxiety by obstetrical providers. *Journal of Women's Health* 19(3):477–490

Green, E.K. Hamshere, M., Forty, L., Gordon-Smith, K., Fraser, C., Russell, E., Grozeva, D., Kirov, G., Holmans, P., Moran, J.L., Purcell, S., Sklar, P., Owen, M.J., O'Donovan, M.C., Jones, L.; WTCCC, Jones, I.R. & Craddock, N. (2013). Replication of bipolar disorder susceptibility alleles and identification of two novel genome-wide significant associations in a new bipolar disorder case-control sample. *Molecular Psychiatry* 18(12):1302–1307

Hanington, L. Heron, J., Stein, A. & Ramchandani, P. (2012). Parental depression and child outcomes – is marital conflict the missing link? *Child Care Health and Development* 38(4):520–529

Henshaw, C. Foreman, D. & Cox, J.L. (2004). Postnatal blues: a risk factor for postnatal depression. *Journal of Psychosomatic Obstetrics & Gynaecology* 25(3–4):267–272

Kim, D. (2009). Psychiatric consultation of patients with hyperemesis gravidarum. *Archives of Women's Mental Health* 12(2):61–67

Mao, Q., Zhu, L. & Su, X. (2011). A comparison of postnatal depression and related factors between Chinese new mothers and fathers. *Journal of Clinical Nursing* 20(5–6):645–652

Markowitz, S., Friedman, M.A. & Arent, S.M. (2008). Understanding the relationship between obesity and depression: Causal mechanisms and implications for treatment. *Clinical Psychology: Science and Practice* V15, N1

Martin, C. (2012). *Perinatal Mental Health A clinical guide.* Cumbria: M&K Publishing

McCarthy, F., Khashan, A., North, R., Moss-Morris, R., Baker, P., Dekker, G., Postonn, L. & Kenny, L.C. (2011). A prospective cohort study investigating associations between hyperemesis gravidarum and cognitive, behavioural and emotional well-being in pregnancy. PLoS ONE 6(11):e27678 doi: 10.1371/journal.pone.0027678

Meltzer-Brody, S. (2014). Treating bipolar disorder in perinatal women when psychiatric hospitalization is necessary: A report from the first U.S. based inpatient perinatal unit. In Abstracts for the International Marce Society for Perinatal Mental Health Biennial Scientific Conference. *Archives of Women's Mental Health* 18(2) published online April 2015

Molyneaux, E., Poston, L., Ashurst-Williams, S. & Howard, L.M. (2014). Obesity and mental disorders during pregnancy and postpartum. A systematic review and meta-analysis. *Obstetrics and Gynecology* 123(4):857–867

Munk-Olsen, T., Munk Laursen, T., Meltzer-Brody, S., Mortensen, P.B. & Jones, I. (2012). Psychiatric disorders with postpartum onset: possible early manifestations of bipolar affective disorders. *Archives of General Psychiatry* 69(4):428–434

National Institute for Health and Care Excellence (NICE) (2007). *Antenatal and Postnatal Mental Health* (CG45). London: National Institute for Health and Care Excellence

Pawlby, S., Sharpe, D., Hay, D. & O'Keane, V. (2008). Postnatal depression and child outcome at 11 years: The importance of accurate diagnosis. *Journal of Affective Disorder* 107:241–245

Petersen, I., Gilbert, R.E., Evans, S.J.W., Man, S.L. & Nazareth, I. (2011). Pregnancy as a major determinant for discontinuation of antidepressants: an analysis of data from the Health Improvement Network. *Journal of Clinical Psychiatry* 72(7):979–985

Rogan, S.C., Payne, J.L. & Meltzer-Brody, S. (2014). Relationship between depressive mood and maternal obesity: implications for postpartum depression. In W. Nicholson & K. Baptiste-Roberts (eds), *Obesity during Pregnancy in Clinical Practice* (pp. 99–120). London: Springer

Rusaka, M. & Rancans, E. (2014). First episode acute and transient psychotic disorder in Latvia: a 6 year follow up study. *Nordic Journal Psychiatry* 68(1):24–29

Schumacher, M., Zubaran, C. & White, G. (2008). Bringing birth-related paternal depression to the fore. *Women and Birth* 21:65–70

Sharma, V., Xie, B., Campbelll, M.K., Penava, D., Hampson, E., Mazmanian, D. & Pope, C.J. (2013). A prospective study of diagnostic conversion of major depressive disorder to bipolar disorder in pregnancy and postpartum. *Bipolar Disorder* 15(6):713–718

Shivakumar, G., Brandon, A., Snell, P., Santiago-Munoz, P., Johnson, N., Trivedi, M. & Freeman, M. (2010). Antenatal depression: A rationale or studying exercise. *Depression and Anxiety* 28:234–242

Sit, D., Rothschild, A., Wisner, K. & Libert M.A. (2006). A review of postpartum psychosis. *Journal of Women's Health* 15(4):352–368

Simmonds, J. Jones, R., Duggan, C. & Hay, D. (2014). The transition to parenthood and the risk of clinically significant mental problems among fathers. In Abstracts for the International Marce Society for Perinatal Mental Health Biennial Scientific Conference. *Archives of Women's Mental Health* 18(2):315 published online April 2015

Stein, A., Woolley, H. & McPherson, K. (1999). Conflict between mothers with eating disorders and their infants during mealtimes. *British Journal of Psychiatry* 175:455–461

Talge, N.M., Neal, C. & Glover, V. (2007). Early Stress, translational research and prevention science network: fetal and neonatal experience on child and adolescent mental health. Antenatal maternal stress and long-term effects on child neurodevelopment: how and why? *Journal of Child Psychology and Psychiatry* 48(34):245–261

Toh, S., Li, Q., Cheetham, T.C., Cooper, W.O., Davis R.L., Dublin, S. Hammad, T.A., Li, D-K, Pawloski, P.A., Pinheiro, S.P., Raebel, M.A., Scott, P.E., Smith, D.H., Bobo, W.V., Lawrence, J.M., Dashevsky, I., Haffenreffer, K., Avalos, L.A. & Andrade, S.E. (2013). Prevalence and trends in the use of antipsychotic medications during pregnancy in the U.S., 2001–2007: a population-based study of 585,615 deliveries. *Archives of Women's Mental Health* 16(2):149–157

WHO (1948). Preamble to the Constitution of the World Health Organization as adopted by the International Health Conference, New York, 19–22 June 1946; signed on 22 July 1946 by the representatives of 61 States (Official Records of the World Health Organization, no. 2, p. 100) and entered into force on 7 April 1948

Wisner, K. *et al.* (2013). Onset timing, thoughts of self-harm, and diagnoses in postpartum women with screen-positive depression findings. *JAMA Psychiatry*. Online vol:1–9

Zelkowitz, P., Saucier, J.F., Wang, T., Katofsky, L., Valenzuela, M. & Westreich, R. (2008). Stability and change in depressive symptoms from pregnancy to two months postpartum in childbearing immigrant women. *Archives of Women's Mental Health* 11(1):1–11

Zimbalidi, C.F., Cantilino, A., Montenegro A.C., Paes, J.A., De Albuquerque, T.L. & Sougey, E.B. (2009). Postpartum obsessive disorder: prevalence, and clinical characteristics. *Comprehensive Psychiatry* 50(6):503–509

THE IMPACT OF PERINATAL MENTAL ILLNESS

2

IMPACT ON THE FOETUS

Research has emphasised the need to pay attention to the demanding stressors that mothers may be subjected to during the pregnancy, as this can have a specific effect not only on the mother, but on her unborn child. If a mother is anxious, stressed or depressed while pregnant, there is an increased risk that her infant may have a broad range of adverse outcomes, which include emotional problems, impaired cognitive development and signs of attention deficit hyperactivity disorder. The situations which would cause stress might include domestic abuse, poverty, war or other traumatic events, some of which may be unavoidable. These findings are important because during pregnancy the female hormones trigger changes in mood.

Recent studies have indicated that the complex influences stress and anxiety have on both the mother and her foetus during pregnancy are precipitated by the hypothalamus, pituitary gland and the adrenal glands. This is known as the hypothalamic, pituitary, adrenal (HPA) axis. If a mother is subjected to stressful situations, corticotrophin releasing hormone (CRH) is produced by the hypothalamus. The CRH stimulates the pituitary to produce adrenocorticotropic hormone (ACTH) which in turn influences the adrenal gland to produce cortisol. The increasing levels of the mother's circulating cortisol stop the production of CRH from her pituitary. The placenta CRH continues the production of the mother's ACTH and further cortisol is produced. The level of cortisol gradually increases during pregnancy, however, high levels of cortisol, produced either in response to an unremittingly distressful situation experienced by the mother, or produced as a response to stress by the foetus, stimulate the placenta to increase the production of CRH. These can rise to toxic levels and are capable of causing the premature delivery of the baby. It is thought that the changes in levels of hormones may then influence the mother's mood making her more anxious, finding it difficult to cope. The neglect of a mother's mood state can have consequences for both her and her infant and therefore it remains important that the mother's well-being is considered in the early stages of pregnancy as well as following the birth of her infant (Talge *et al.* 2007, Glover 2014).

IMPACT ON THE MOTHER

Often depression is described as a mild to moderate non-psychotic illness characterised by persistent and pervasive symptoms which have a significant effect on day-to-day life. These include a loss of pleasure, indicating the mother may not have the joy of being a mother, just when she needs joy the most. A persistent low mood can rob a mother of her energy, resulting in tiredness, which is not improved by her inability to enjoy quality, undisturbed sleep. This may be caused by her own emotional state rather than the demands of her infant.

A further cardinal feature of depression is psychomotor retardation (Parker et al. 1995). This results in the slowing down of the mother's thought processes, whereby emotional reactions are sluggish, measured and deliberate and may be interpreted as disinterest or indifference. This impairs the mother's concentration, and her memory may also be affected, making it difficult to remember and retain instructions, or to remember appointments. There is also a reduction in any physical activity requiring significant motivation and effort to complete domestic and other chores. This inability to perform in a productive way can lead the mother to feelings of self-reproach and guilt, culminating in fault and blame. It is not uncommon for these emotions to lead to the feelings of inadequacy which may ultimately result in suicidal thoughts.

Mothers whose infants have developed a pattern for waking frequently and for prolonged periods throughout the night have a greater risk of developing depressive symptoms. However, the mother's ability to sleep increases once there is improvement in the infant's sleep pattern (Hildebrandt & Young 2007, Okun et al. 2011). Although this research remains limited, there is a lack of national guidance and provision available for families struggling with serious sleep deprivation and the sequelae from this on their mental health and relationships. Sleep difficulties are one of the commonest reasons why health workers are consulted and therefore it is essential that the advice they give parents is consistent and evidenced based (Fisher 2013).

Along with poor sleep patterns, compromised nutrition is problematic. The demands of pregnancy, motherhood and lactation cause significant nutritional stress on the woman's body. Good nutrition is essential for optimum brain function, which is responsible for every decision and action made. Studies have shown that a poor diet, caused by irregular meals or easy to prepare, satisfying foods high in carbohydrates or salts, has an adverse effect on mood. Dietary deficiencies in selenium, iron, zinc and vitamin B12 were found to be more common in depressed mothers than those who were not depressed (Bodnar & Wisner 2005). A poor intake of omega 3 fatty acid, found in fish oil, has been shown to increase the probability of depression (He et al. 2008), while a deficiency in folate reduces the response to antidepressants.

LIBIDO

The self-limiting nature of pregnancy and early childbirth has a naturally disruptive impact on sexual desires. The physical changes and progressive increase in size, both internally and externally, make posture difficult and sexual activity challenging for the woman. Little attention has been paid by researchers to couples' sexuality, sensuality and intimacy during and after the pregnancy. In a study by de Montigny *et al.* (2014), it was found that from the pregnancy to the postpartum period, couples identified various challenges in maintaining a satisfactory sexual life. These challenges affected the marital relationship, to the point that some feared partner infidelity. Studies have suggested that sexual intimacy has the capacity to improve the mood of depressed mothers, which encouraged the women to initiate sexual relations. It was postulated that women construct their sexuality to cope with their distress. Two thirds of women are affected by hyperemesis and ptyalism, the compounding factors which affect intimate behaviour (Annagur 2013).

SUICIDE

Suicide accounts for one in twenty deaths both during pregnancy and postnatally. Some studies have found that many of the women who die by suicide are often from low income areas. Over the last two decades, along with cardiac disease and infections, perinatal mental illness has been a leading cause of maternal death, contributing to 15 per cent of all maternal deaths in pregnancy and during the first six months postnatally. In a study by Munk-Olsen *et al.* (2014) results indicated that mothers with postnatal mental illness have a considerably better long-term survival than other female psychiatric patients without children. Generally mothers with psychiatric disorders, regardless of timing of onset, had lower mortality rates than psychiatric patients without children. However, mothers with postnatal mental illness are three times more likely to die compared with the population of healthy mothers (CMACE 2011).

Pervading thoughts include the dread of facing the day, to thoughts that the world would be better off without them. Women are often overwhelmed by feelings of unhappiness until the only recourse is to plummet downwards, becoming so depressed that the mother decides her own fate and attempts to extricate herself from life, often permanently (Cox *et al.* 1987, Oates 2003, Patrick 2013).

Suicide may occur during pregnancy but there is little indication that pregnancy itself is the main motivation and it has been associated with a lower risk of suicide. Following birth, however, one protective factor is the dependent infant (Marzuk *et al.* 1997). The exception is in bipolar disorder where, as part of the reactivation of the disorder, suicide may emerge as the pregnancy progresses. Deliberate self-harm appears to have a similar prevalence in both pregnant and non-pregnant women.

Opinion is divided on the morality of the act, debating whether the mother is abandoning her infant for selfish reasons or abdicating from the responsibilities to allow someone more capable to care for the infant. Women appear to be neither seeking attention nor seeking help, but calculating and intentionally choosing their death. The woman with a terminal illness will have enduring support, but the woman who 'chooses' her own fate, albeit determined by a mental illness, has little sympathy. If this mindset were altered, there might be further research into treating the terminal decline of depression.

DOMESTIC ABUSE

Women with depression during the perinatal period were found to be three times more likely to have been the victims of domestic violence and five times more likely to have experienced it while pregnant (Flach *et al.* 2011). During the years 2006–08, thirty-nine (12 per cent) of the women who died had features of domestic abuse. For eight of these women, murdered by their husband or partner, the abuse was fatal. Three other women were murdered by non-family members. Many of the other women, who died from a range of other causes, had proactively self-reported domestic abuse to a health care professional either before or during their pregnancy (CMACE 2011). The lack of knowledge on how to manage this condition often increased their frustration, highlighting the fact that asking questions about any incidence of domestic violence should not be avoided (Rodrigues *et al.* 2008, Howard & Feder 2013).

STIGMA

Stigma refers to the lack of awareness and knowledge of perinatal mental health and the attitudes towards mentally ill parents, which can culminate in prejudice. The behaviour of the individual and society can lead to discrimination against the parents which may disenfranchise them, leaving them socially disadvantaged (Thornicroft *et al.* 2008).

Writers have likened mental illness to a social deviance which disqualifies people from social acceptance. This is primarily because of their ineffectiveness in society and demands on the health service. The unpredictability of severe mental illness also makes them a threat to social order. This opinion was reinforced by the fact that it was once believed that madness is contagious and people were best housed in asylums away from communities. The origin of the word 'asylum' served as a retreat or refuge. The beliefs may have moderated but there remains a steadfast prejudice and shaping of public opinion against those who fail to comply with society's accepted regimes.

Maternal mental illness is no longer considered in isolation, and increasingly the needs and involvement of the father/partner are recognised. There are complex, cross-partner associations with the quality of the relationship and the depressive symptoms in both mothers and fathers. In studies, fathers have suggested that sometimes they felt marginalised and avoided confrontation with health workers, as often they were made to feel responsible for the condition of their partner and were perturbed at their inability to make it better for her. The demands of society suggest that men should provide the protective armour for the family (Conde *et al.* 2011, Gilligan *et al.* 2011). The worried father often colluded with the mother to minimise the effect of stigma and the threat of having the child 'taken away', which is a familiar fear reiterated throughout the literature (Netmums 2012, 4children 2011). It was found that often the health worker neglected to seek the father's opinion and relied solely on the views of the mother to make a judgement, thus compounding the father's feelings of being marginalised.

Wynter *et al.* (2014) found that rather than insufficient affection or care, the dimension of intimate relationship, which involved being critical and coercive, was most strongly associated with emotional well-being. There is significant research which suggests the importance of enriching the partner relationship, as couples approach parenthood, to offset the profound impact of a new baby on the dynamics of the relationship and on the couple's own perinatal mental health (Ayers *et al.* 2014, Kerstis *et al.* 2014).

The resulting factors which can arise from parental perinatal mental illness are varied in number and intensity making it a significant public health concern.

IMPACT ON THE INFANT

During the infant's early months, the mother, in particular is his main source of motivation, offering highly arousing and visually stimulating communication forms, to shape his immature brain. This facilitates both his social and cognitive development, which is imperative for his healthy maturity. Numerous studies have shown that some depressed mothers provide distorted environments for their infants (Collett 2005, Goodman *et al.* 2011, Wynter *et al.* 2014). Some may be overwhelmed with the responsibility of care required by the infant and over compensate by indulging in the infant's basic needs by excessive feeding or being over protective of his safety. Attempting to achieve this level of attainment often leads to feelings of guilt and inadequacy. The florid symptoms of depression may penalise the depressed mother as she may find it difficult to engage with her infant. If she feels little joy or is unable to smile at her infant, the positive effect of stimulating the release of hormones and neurotransmitters – dopamine, catecholamine, adrenaline and other neuro peptides within the brain, which are responsible for increased alertness and memory and allows the facilitation of the learning process – is damaged (Chiarello 2010).

The mother with depressive symptoms may be overwhelmed with the complexities of poor self-esteem, low expectations and other negative emotions and may lack high reflective functioning which prevents the ability to see her infant as a separate, autonomous individual and cannot attribute the emotions, thoughts, feelings and desires to her child, and is therefore unable to differentiate and separate them from her own emotions and desires. Without this capacity, the parent–child relationship is weakened and the infant fails to learn how to understand and regulate his behaviour, which in turn fails to support the infant's cognitive development. This inability to respond empathetically results in the depressed mother having an impaired relationship with her infant. She is insensitive to the infant's cues and the complex process of mutual regulation. There is an interference with any positive maternal–infant interaction and the process of secure attachment is disrupted, which is associated with the infant's poor social interactions and lower cognitive development when older.

The research has uncovered that the emotional needs of the child himself are unmet if the mother struggles with her own needs. This can lead to many outcomes which can include lack of attachment, containment, where the baby feels safe, and the dance of reciprocity, where the mother finds it difficult to tune into the infant's cues and needs (Murray *et al.* 1996, Paulson *et al.* 2006, Ramchandani *et al.* 2008, Pawlby *et al.* 2008, Sethna *et al.* 2012, Barker 2013).

Paternal depression has been associated with a poor sense of coherence with their infant. The father may be less attentive towards the infant, with negative behaviours, speech often critical and tending more towards spanking rather than reading (Davis *et al.* 2011, Kerstis *et al.* 2013, Parfitt *et al.* 2013).

Taking the outcomes a stage further and considering the future of the child, if there is no intervention to improve the mental health of the mother, father and the child, there is a chance that the child's intellectual development will be compromised leading to difficulties with schooling and probably poor attendance and attainment. The poor cognitive development may lead to behavioural issues, with poor routine, structures or boundaries, and difficulties in forming relationships and interactions with others. This may ultimately lead to anxiety and/or depression within the child.

IMPACT ON SOCIETY

The recognition, management and treatment of perinatal mental illness should be crucial throughout the world. It is not solely about the impact on the individual or family but the collective outcomes for society. Infants born to depressed mothers may be disenfranchised of the prerequisites of life which enable them to succeed. This in turn has an impact on future generations, particularly those who already reside in impoverished societies who need to have the emotional as well as physical well-being to improve their societal outcomes.

The initial signs of a depressive disorder may be difficult to detect as often parents are skilful at disguising how they really feel; however, with an increased awareness of the symptoms of perinatal mental disorders or illness, the health worker should be able to observe physical and behavioural changes, if not psychological ones. The intuitive health worker, who is familiar with the parent, might notice a change in appearance – that the parent is 'not their usual self'. Outward appearances might not reflect how they dressed prior to the pregnancy or the birth of the infant. The mother's make-up may be minimal or absent, hair not brushed or unkempt. The pace and movements might be noticeably sluggish or deliberate, and body shape may have changed because of an increase or decrease in weight. The changes or lack of attachment in the parent–infant reaction are also indicators to cause concern. The outlined factors will, hopefully, help the health worker to have a deeper understanding of the impact and influences of perinatal mental disorders on the father, infant and society, highlighting the need for support and assurance. This can only be achieved by asking the questions and listening.

REFERENCES

4Children (2011). *Suffering in Silence.* www.4children.org

Annagur, B. (2013). Do psychiatric disorders continue during pregnancy in women with hyperemesis gravidarum: a prospective study. *General Hospital Psychiatry* 35:492–496

Ayers, S., Jessup, D., Pike, A., Parfitt, Y. & Ford, E. (2014). The role of adult attachment style, birth intervention and support in posttraumatic stress after childbirth: A prospective study. *Journal of Affective Disorders* 155:295–298

Barker, E. (2013). The duration and timing of maternal depression as a moderator of the relationship between dependent interpersonal stress, contextual risk and early child dysregulation. *Psychological Medicine* 43(8):1587–1596

Bodnar, L. & Wisner, K. (2005). Nutrition and depression: Implications for improving mental health among childbearing-aged women. *Biological Psychiatry* 58(9):679–685

Centre for Maternal and Child Enquiries (CMACE) (2011). Saving Mothers' Lives: reviewing maternal deaths to make motherhood safer: 2006–08. *The Eighth Report on Confidential Enquiries into Maternal Deaths in the United Kingdom.* BJOG 118 (Suppl. 1):1–203

Chiarello, M. (2010). Humor as a teaching tool. *Journal of Psychology Nursing* 48(8):35–41

Conde, A., Figueiredo, B. & Bifulco, A. (2011). Attachment style and psychological adjustment in couples. *Attachment & Human Development* 13 (3):271–291

Collett, J.L. (2005). What kind of mother am I? Impression management and the social construction of motherhood. *Symbolic Interaction* 28:327–347

Cox, J. L., Holden, J.M. & Sagovsky, R. (1987). Detection of postnatal depression. Development of the 10-item Edinburgh Postnatal Depression Scale. *British Journal of Psychiatry* 150:782–786

Davis, N.R., Davis, M.M., Freed, G.L. & Clark, S.J. (2011). Fathers' depression related to positive and negative parenting behaviors with 1-year-old children. *PEDIATRICS* 127(4):612–618

De Montigny, F., de Montigny-Gauthier, P. & Dennie-Fillion, E. (2014). La sexualité après la naissance et en contexte d'allaitement maternel: expérience des mères et des pères. In C. Bayard et C. Chouinard (eds), *La promotion de l'allaitement maternel au Québec: Regards critiques* (pp. 137–158). Montréal: Les Éditions du Remue-ménage

Fisher, M. (2013). Sleep matters for health visitors: evidence and best practice. *Nursing in Practice, Health Visitor Supplement* May/June

Flach, C., Leese, M., Heron, J., Evans, J., Feder, G., Sharp, D. & Howard, L. (2011). Antenatal domestic violence, maternal mental health and subsequent child behaviour: A cohort study. *Bjog – an International Journal of Obstetrics and Gynaecology* 118(11):1383–1391

Gilligan, P., Manby, M. & Pickburn, C. (2011). Fathers' involvement in children's services: Exploring local and national issues in 'Moorlandstown'. *British Journal of Social Work Advance Access* published online 26 May 2011

Glover, V. (2014). Maternal depression, anxiety and stress during pregnancy and child outcome; what needs to be done. Best Practice & Research. *Clinical Obstetrics & Gynaecology* 28:25

Goodman, S.H., Rouse, M.H., Connell, A.M., Broth, M.R., Hall, C.M. & Heyward, D. (2011). Maternal depression and child psychopathology: A meta-analytic review. *Clinical Child and Family Psychology Review* 14:1–27

He, K., Lio, K., Daviglus, M.L. *et al.* (2008). Intakes of long-chain n-3 poly-unsaturated fatty acids and fish in relation to measurements of subclinical atherosclerosis. *American Journal of Clinical Nutrition* 88(4):1111–1118

Hildebrandt, K. & Young, M. (2007). Night waking in 6-month-old infants and maternal depressive symptoms. *Journal of Applied Developmental Psychology* 28(5–6):493–498

Howard, L. & Feder, G. (2013). *Domestic Violence and Mental Health*. London: RCPsych Publication

Kerstis, B., Engstrom, G., Edlund, B. & Aarts, C. (2013). Association between mothers' and fathers' depressive symptoms, sense of coherence and perception of their child's temperament in early parenthood in Sweden. *Scandinavian Journal of Public Health* 41(3):233–239

Kerstis, B., Berglund, A., Engstrom, G., Edlund, N., Sylven, S. & Aarts, C. (2014). Depressive symptoms postpartum among parents are associated with marital separation: A Swedish cohort study. *Scandinavian Journal of Public Health* published online 22 July 2014 DOI: 10.1177/1403494814542262:1–9

Marzuk, P.M., Tardiff, K. Leon, A.C., Hirsch, C.S., Portera, L., Hartwell, N. & Iqbal, M.I. (1997). Lower risk of suicide during pregnancy. *American Journal of Psychiatry* 154(1):122–123

Munk-Olsen, T., Munk Laursen, T., Meltzer-Brody, S., Mortensen, P.O. & Jones, I. (2012). Psychiatric disorders with postpartum onset: possible early manifestations of bipolar affective disorders. *Archives of General Psychiatry* 69(4):428–434

Munk-Olsen, T., Jones, I. & Laursen, T.M. (2014). Birth order and postpartum psychiatric disorders. *Bipolar Disorder*. May, 16(3):300-3007. doi: 10.1111/bdi.12145. Epub 31 October 2013

Murray, L., Fiori-Cowley, A., Hooper, R. & Cooper, P. (1996). The impact of postnatal depression and associated adversity on early mother-infant interactions and later infant outcome. *Child Development* 67:2512–2526

Netmums (2012). *Antenatal and postnatal depression*. www.netmums.com

Oates, M. (2003). Perinatal psychiatric disorders: a leading cause of maternal morbidity and mortality. *British Medical Bulletin* 67:219–229

Okun, M., Luther, J., Prather, A., Perel, J., Wisniewski, S., Sit, D., Prairie, B.A. & Wisner, K. (2011). Changes in sleep quality, but not hormones predict time to postpartum depression recurrence. *Journal of Affective Disorders* 130(3):378–384

Parfitt, Y., Pike, A. & Ayers, S. (2013). The impact of parents' mental health on parent-baby interaction: A prospective study. *Infant Behavior and Development* 36(4):599–608

Parker, D., Hadzi-Pavlovic, D., Hickie, I, Austin, M.P., Mitchell, P., Wilhelm, K., Hickie, I., Boyce, P. & Eyers, K. (1995). Sub-typing depression I. Is psychomotor disturbance necessary and sufficient to the definition of melancholia? *Psychological Medicine* 25:815–823

Patrick, K. (2013). It's time to put maternal suicide under the microscope. *CMAJ* DOI:10.1503/cmaj.131248

Paulson, J.F., Dauber, S. & Leiferman, J.A. (2006). Individual and combined effects of postpartum depression in mothers and fathers on parenting behavior. *Pediatrics* 118 (2):659–668

Pawlby, S., Sharp, D., Hay, D.F. & O'Keane, V. (2008). Postnatal depression and child outcome at 11 years: The importance of accurate diagnosis. *Journal of Affective Disorders* 107:241–245

Ramchandani, P., O'Connor, T.G., Evans, J., Heron, J., Murray, L. & Stein, A. (2008). Depression in men in the postnatal period and later child psycho-pathology: A population cohort study. *Journal of American Academy of Child and Adolescent Psychiatry* 47(4):390–398

Rodrigues, T., Roche, L. & Barros, H. (2008). Physical abuse during pregnancy and preterm delivery. *AJOG* 198:171–174

Sethna, V., Murray, L., Ramchandani, P. & Press, C. (2012). Depressed fathers' speech to their 3-month-old infants: A study of cognitive and mentalizing features in paternal speech. *Psychological Medicine* 42(11):2361–2371

Talge, N.M., Neal, C. & Glover, V. (2007). Early stress, translational research and prevention science network: Fetal and neonatal experience on child and adolescent mental health. Antenatal maternal stress and long-term effects on child neurodevelopment: how and why? *Journal of Child Psychology & Psychiatry* 48(34):245–261

Thornicroft, G., Brohan, E., Kassam, A. & Lewis- Holmes, E. (2008). Reducing stigma and discrimination: Candidate interventions. *International Journal of Mental Health Systems* 2:3

Wynter, K., Rowe, H.J. & Fisher, J. (2014). Interactions between perceptions of relationship quality and postnatal depressive symptoms in Australian, primiparous women and their partners. *Australian Journal of Primary Health* 20:174–181

3

ASSESSMENT AND TRAINING

ASSESSMENT

Health workers concerned with maternal health need to encompass both the emotional and mental health of the mother as a composite part of the holistic assessment (Brown and Bacigalupo 2006, Morrell *et al.* 2011). During a systematic review of psychosocial and psychological interventions, conducted by Dennis (2005), it was found that individual interventions which were targeted at mothers who were at risk in the postnatal period, were beneficial. Various studies have recognised the role of the health visitor as fundamental in detecting postnatal depression and other maternal mood disorders (Hanley 2009, Morrell *et al.* 2011). Their communication skills, immediacy to the mother, ability to detect postnatal depression and develop a rapport, make them one of the more appropriate health workers to invite the mother to become involved within a therapeutic intervention. To assist with this process, the competent use of the appropriate screening tools and clinical assessment of the mother's mood can help to verify how she is feeling. This will facilitate the necessary treatments or social support to assist the mother to return to a state of sound emotional well-being. Sensitive detection with appropriate questions allows the mother to explore, understand her feelings and ultimately solve or alleviate her own problems.

EDINBURGH POSTNATAL DEPRESSION SCALE (EPDS)

Currently the EPDS is the most validated and utilised self-reporting measurement in the world. It provides a useful tool to help assess the mother's mood (Cox *et al.* 1987). The EPDS has proven to be an effective diagnostic tool, although its sensitivity, specificity and predictive power depends on chosen cut-off scores (Appleby *et al.* 1994, Beck & Gable 2001, Wylie *et al.* 2011). A score of 10 or more is indicative of depression and it is probable that a mother who scores above 13 is likely to be suffering from a depressive disorder of varying degrees. The maximum score is 30. The United Kingdom NICE guidelines currently do not recommend using routine assessments such as

EPDS because it is not cost effective. However Austin *et al.* (2011, 2013) demonstrate the benefits of this, showing how maternal mental health improved because of routine screening.

Despite controversial arguments about its use during the past twelve years, the EPDS has few rivals. Practitioners are advised to adhere to the suggestion by the National Screening Committee (UK) that any proposal that the EPDS is a diagnostic tool is avoided and that it is used in conjunction with a deeper assessment of the mother's mood before a clinical decision is made.

The global acceptance of the EPDS is emphasised by the abundance of studies which have examined the efficacy and reliability of the scoring system. A comprehensive assessment of the studies which have been validated, and those which have not, can be found in a Western Australian document (DoH GWA 2006). Health workers have determined the usefulness of the tool and generally felt that this enabled the focus to shift solely from the infant, to now include the mother–infant relationship.

The early detection of postnatal depression and the implementation of direct, appropriate evidence based interventions is recommended by the NICE Guidelines (2007). There are many conflicting accounts of the most appropriate screening tool, and psychotherapeutic intervention; however it would appear that when the recovery rate is compared with the absence of any intervention, each individual approach has merit.

Since the introduction of the NICE Guidelines for Antenatal and Postnatal Mental Health, another assessment process, the Whooley Questions, clearly focuses on the DSM-1V criteria for a depressive disorder. The following two questions are asked by the health worker:

> During the past month, have you often been bothered by feeling down, depressed, or hopeless?

and

> During the past month, have you often been bothered by little interest or pleasure in doing things?

A positive answer to the two questions determines whether a mother has depressive symptoms, whereas any negative responses make the diagnosis of depression highly unlikely. It has been suggested that the questions are asked by prime health workers to mothers who are at high risk of, or who present with, symptoms which are suggestive of depression. The questions provide the opportunity to screen without the need for a formal assessment (Whooley *et al.* 1997).

The wide use of the Whooley Questions by general practitioners in the UK has encouraged some health workers to adopt the same process for continuity of care. However there is a danger that this too can become a tick-box exercise, whereby once the mother has answered the questions either positively or negatively, the health worker might feel the process of assessment has been completed. A similar criticism has been levied at the use of the EPDS and previous reports have been unfavourable of its use, suggesting that reliance on the answers damages the intuitive experiences of the practitioner (Barker 1998). The definitive score or response from the Whooley Questions may set a course of action which is reliant on other types of treatment, rather than utilising the existing knowledge and skills of the health professional. Although there is no definite research, anecdotal evidence suggests that screening for depression using a screening tool as well as intuition, is not universal within the UK.

THE PATIENT HEALTH QUESTIONNAIRE 9 (PHQ9)

This questionnaire is based on the diagnostic criteria for major depressive disorder in the Diagnostic and Statistical Manual Fifth Edition (DSM-V). It consists of two components: to assess the symptoms and the functional impairment. These ascertain whether the mother has signs of depression. It gives a baseline score on to which the management and treatment may be underpinned. When it is repeated it can help to monitor the progress of the mother following the interventions.

The PHQ 9 may be used as part of a telephone conversation. It is proposed it is used as an *aide memoire* to help the health worker cover all likely aspects of the mother's lifestyle. For example, the question about 'appetite' can generate discussion about the mother's eating habits and patterns. However, if the mother has an eating disorder the question may be seen as ambiguous as the mother may not see her appetite as being particularly worrying.

Whatever assessment tool is used, it is important to remember that it is not the score that matters but the holistic assessment, using the knowledge about perinatal mental disorders and the impact they will have on the mother and her family to make a judgement on the parent's mood and the potential well-being of the family.

LIMITATIONS OF SELF-REPORT SCALES

The format in which the form is introduced to the mother is important, ensuring the mother does not regard it as a test or diagnosis. It should be carried out with clarity and sensitivity. It should be explained that high scoring does not necessarily mean poor parenting or that any significant action needs to be taken (Seeley 2001). Honesty should be paramount as several instances have been recorded where the forms have been falsified to avoid imagined detrimental consequences, for example, the infant 'being taken into care' or the involvement of social services. There are debates about the exact location where the mother should fill in the form and the ideal place is in the home, but with time restrictions this is not always feasible.

As the questions are completed by the mother there is the risk that she might exaggerate or understate the answers to the questions. Training to help interpret the questionnaire should eliminate any discrepancies about the way in which the questions are answered. With careful explanation, the health worker can help the mother to understand how she may have misinterpreted a particular question.

Language difficulties are another consideration. The EPDS has been translated into over fifty languages making the availability more accessible for geographically diverse and non-English speaking mothers.

Some features of the screening questionnaires do not focus on the mother's sleep pattern, enjoyment of her infant, appetite habits or concentration. An important adage is the determination of her ideations of previous self-harm or suicidal intentions and acknowledging the depth of these thoughts and feelings. Equipped with the knowledge of the mother's mental health and the impact it has on her daily living and her relationship with her infant, it is possible to offer listening visits as an intervention.

LISTENING VISITS AS AN INTERVENTION

Many mothers have reported they did not have the insight to be able to recognise their depressive symptoms or were aware of the stigma that any confession would produce. Therefore they did not actively seek help. Systematic screening, both with the use of the EPDS and/or Whooley Questions, and the deeper exploration of the mother's mood, with the use of appropriate questioning in the clinical interview, can help to establish the characteristics of an existing or developing depression.

There is the assumption that listening is an easy task which can be successfully achieved by anyone. It is sometimes questioned what would be difficult about this, and it has been suggested that listening is an innate skill that everyone is capable of. However, although humans have the ability to listen, whether they do it properly is arguable. The process is largely dependent on the empathy expressed by the listener. The philosophy of just listening can be a daunting task for some health workers as it contravenes the need for prescriptive interventions. Most health workers, as facilitators, operate to resolve or repair problems and there might be a tendency to offer solutions. It is a skilled task which relies on time and patience to achieve.

BENEFITS OF LISTENING VISITS

The benefit of the listening visit is that it can successfully be delivered in the home situation. This negates the need for childcare arrangements or transport, which is of particular importance in rural or socio-economically deprived areas. It is planned, time limited and focused. The person-centred approach ensures the ability for the rapport to develop and the contracted time between the mother and the health worker ensures mutual compliance. As the process takes place around the time of childbirth the visit has the ability to optimise the parent's relationship with the infant. The health worker's case load may include rural areas where access to the specialist perinatal services may be limited or non-existent, or densely populated suburban areas where psychiatric services may be restricted. The confident and competent health worker, in perinatal mental health, has the ability to manage and improve detection of depressive disorders and to understand the limitations of that process.

Sometimes listening can be frustrating and health workers feel that they are not progressing or become 'stuck' in the therapeutic relationship. They may feel the parent is not improving as quickly as expected or that the mother is becoming too dependent on the health worker's interventions. This can make health workers doubt their own abilities. Training can provide the practitioner with the skills and knowledge to detect and manage perinatal mental health disorders, but a basic requirement is the provision of good support and supervision.

TRAINING

Morrell *et al.* (2011) demonstrated the necessity of specialised training for health visitors. Two groups of health visitors, one group trained in the assessment of postnatal depression and either cognitive behavioural therapies or listening techniques, the other group with no specialist training, were individually assigned to mothers who were at risk of developing a depressive disorder. The study found that mothers were less likely to become depressed if their health visitor has undergone additional training in listening visits or basic cognitive behavioural techniques. They were compared with mothers who did not receive this care and it was found that these mothers were more likely to develop depression six months following the birth of their infant.

This has supported the findings of previous studies which acknowledge the efficacy of health visitor intervention (Holden 1996) and that individual non-directive counselling is effective (O'Hara *et al.* 2000, Alder and Truman 2002, Dennis 2005). Listening visits are effective in treating mild to moderate depression. When Holden *et al.* (1989) first evaluated the impact of listening visits, it was found that 68 per cent of depressed mothers who received the listening visits recovered compared with 38 per cent in the control group. Subsequent studies have replicated these findings (Cooper *et al.* 2003, Morrell *et al.* 2009). Intervening with psychological interventions offers a workable alternative to help mothers overcome postnatal depression.

The first accepted form of training in the listening visit was done by Sandra Elliott *et al.* (2001) and Gerrard *et al.* (1993) who trained health visitors in the detection, treatment and prevention of postnatal depression, the use of the EPDS, and gave information about the value and practice of non-directive counselling and about preventative strategies. Despite the passage of time, often there is the assumption that because some health workers are trained to have the resilience to offer expertise and often prescriptive solutions in individual interventions in childcare, they are also capable of developing therapeutic interventions with mothers who have mental health issues. Theoretically this is true, but often mental ill health and other disorders are not addressed in any significant depth during some pre- and post-registration training programmes.

A report by Adams (2008) found that there were considerable regional disparities in the preparation of health visitors to address mental health issues. It was found that in an audit survey the number of health visitors who were able to access training during 2007 averaged 35 per cent in London, while in the South West it was only 16 per cent. However, in 2013, health visitor 'perinatal mental health champions' were trained in England, with the vision that all of the health visitors in England would have some training in perinatal mental health and listening visits (iHV 2014). The lack of a recognised national curriculum means that practitioners have often sought training by other routes, sometimes within the private sector. The training courses vary in duration, depending on the current knowledge of the practitioner. To suggest that mental health issues can be taught within a short rigid time framework is tantamount to implying that all the issues around heart disease, for instance, can be learnt within a prescribed timeframe.

The implementation of the listening visit is defined by building on the existing communication skills of the practitioner, who should also have a sound knowledge, not only of the aetiology, but the physiological and social impact of perinatal mental health. The completion of the EPDS or a similar assessment tool, is the precursor to a listening programme. The health worker should be competent in the use of an assessment tool and acquainted with the guidelines for its implementation (Seeley *et al.* 1996, Seeley 2001, Cox and Holden 2003). Training in the interpretation of the clinical interview and mood assessment encourages the practitioner to increase and develop their active reflective listening skills.

The detection of and attempts to prevent mental illness is an integral part of health. Research has shown the importance of the impact of good mental health on the whole family's emotional, spiritual and physical well-being. Early awareness of and intervention in mental health disorders can prevent the mother's mood from deteriorating and that can only have positive outcomes for the mother, father and the family. The intrinsic skills of practice will qualify health workers to be naturally disposed to the appropriate requirements of psychological approaches. The training helps to develop and expand their existing abilities.

When prioritising of the work analysis of staff, the management needs to determine the overall benefits of mental health treatment during the ante- and postnatal periods. However, despite overwhelming evidence to suggest that early intervention is essential to ensure the effects on the family are minimised, it is probable that the labour-intense treatment programme, coupled with the need for educational resources and training, often supersedes the more pressing and popular necessities of public health issues.

REFERENCES

Adams, C. (2008). Health visitors are key to the infant mental health agenda – but how well prepared are they? Holding the baby in mind: a public health approach to safeguarding. NSPCC *Conference proceedings*, 26 September, London

Alder, E. & Truman, J. (2002). Counselling for postnatal depression in the voluntary sector. *Psychology and Psychotherapy* 75:207–220

Appleby, L., Gregoire, A., Platz, C., Prince, M. & Kumar, R. (1994). Screening women for high risk of postnatal depression. *Journal of Psychosomatic Research* 38:539–545

Austin, M.P., Middleton, P., Reilly, N. & Highet, N. (2011). Detection and management of mood disorders in the maternity setting: The Australian Clinical Practice Guidelines. *Women and Birth* 26:2–9

Austin, M.P. & Hanley, J. (2013). Perinatal psychosocial assessment and depression screening. *Journal of Health Visiting* 1(10):550

Barker, W. (1998). Let's trust our instincts. *Community Practitioner* 71(9) September 305

Beck, C. & Gable, R. (2001). Further validation of the postpartum depression screening scale. *Nursing Research and Practice* 50:155–164

Brown, H. & Bacigalupo, R. (2006). Health visitors and postnatal depression: identification and practice. *Community Practitioner* 79(2):49–52

Cooper, P.J., Murray, L., Wilson, A. & Romaniuk, H. (2003). Controlled trial of the short- and long-term effect of psychological treatment of post-partum depression. I. Impact on maternal mood. *British Journal of Psychiatry* May 182:412–419

Cox, J. L., Holden, J.M. & Sagovsky, R. (1987). Detection of postnatal depression. Development of the 10-item Edinburgh Postnatal Depression Scale. *British Journal of Psychiatry* 150:782–786

Cox, J. & Holden, J. (2003). *Perinatal Mental Health: A Guide to the Edinburgh Postnatal Depression Scale (EPDS)*. London: Gaskell

Dennis, C.L. (2005). Psychosocial and psychological interventions for prevention of postnatal depression: systematic review. *BMJ* 331(7507):15

Department of Health, Government of Western Australia (2006). *Edinburgh Postnatal Depression Scale (EPDS): Translated Versions – Validated*. Perth, Western Australia: State Perinatal Mental Health Reference Group

Elliot, S.A., Gerrard, J., Ashton, C. & Cox, J. (2001). Training health visitors to reduce levels of depression after childbirth: An evaluation. *Journal of Mental Health* 10(6):613–625

Gerrard, J. Holden J.M., Elliott, S.A., McKenzie, P., McKenzie, J. & Cox, J.L. (1993). A trainer's perspective of an innovative programme teaching health visitors about the detection, treatment and prevention of postnatal depression. *Journal of Advanced Nursing* 18(11):1825–1832

Hanley, J. (2009). *Perinatal Mental Health*. Oxford: Wiley Blackwell

Holden, J. (1996). The role of health visitors in postnatal depression. *International Review of Psychiatry* 8:79–86

Holden, J.M., Sagovsky, R. & Cox, J.L. (1989). Counselling in a general practice setting: Controlled study of health visitor intervention in treatment of postnatal depression. *BMJ* 298:223–226

Institute of Health Visiting (iHV) (2014). *Perinatal Mental Health Champions*. www.ihv.org

Morrell, J., Slade, P., Warner, R., Paley, G., Dixon, S., Walters, S.J., Brugha, T., Barkham, M., Parry, G.J. & Nicholl, J. (2009). Clinical effectiveness of health visitor training in psychologically informed approaches for depression in postnatal women pragmatic cluster randomised trial in primary care. *BMJ* 338(7689):276–280

Morrell, C.J., Ricketts, T., Williams, K., Curran, J. & Barkham, M. (2011). Training health visitors in cognitive behavioural and person-centred approaches for depression in postnatal women as part of a cluster randomised trial and economic evaluation in primary care: the PoNDER trial. *Primary Health Care Research and Development* 12(1):11–20

National Institute for Health and Care Excellence (2007). *Antenatal and Postnatal Mental Health* (CG45). London: National Institute for Health and Care Excellence

O'Hara, M.W., Stuart, S. & Gorman, W.L.L. (2000). Efficacy of interpersonal psychotherapy for postpartum depression. *Archives of General Psychiatry* 57:1039

Seeley, S. (2001). Strengths and limitations of the Edinburgh Postnatal Depression Scale. *CPHVA Conference Proceedings*, October: 16–19

Seeley, S., Murray, L. & Cooper, P. J. (1996). The outcome for mothers and babies of health visitor intervention. *Health Visitor* 69(4):135–138

Whooley, M.A., Avins, A.L., Miranda, J. & Browner, W.S. (1997). Case-finding instruments for depression. Two questions are as good as many. *Journal of General Internal Medicine* 12(7):439–445

Wylie., L., Hollins Martin, C.J., Marland, G., Martin, C.R. & Rankin, J. (2011). The enigma of postnatal depression. *Journal of Psychiatric and Mental Health Nursing* 18:48–58

LISTENING SKILLS AND KNOWLEDGE

4

- How is a listening visit done?
- What skills are a prerequisite?
- Complex approaches
- Challenges

WHAT IS A LISTENING SKILL?

Listening visits are based on the logical and pragmatic clinical theories of Carl Rogers (1957) and provide the basis for a broad application. Rogers recognised that when his clients felt that their views were being acknowledged, accepted, encouraged and not judged, they thrived emotionally. This environment provided the fertile ground to enable the client to become engaged, which in turn, hastened the process of their recovery. Rogers termed this as a 'positive self-regard' and may be interpreted as having confidence in their own positive self esteem. Rogers also recognised the power of these attributes or skills within the listener, and how a fragile and complex relationship might be damaged by an unguarded movement, thought or word from the therapist, which might ultimately lead to a dysfunctional relationship.

Sometimes circumstances govern the type of encouragement that might be presented. Rogers argued that powerful conditions had the ability to fracture beliefs, which might ultimately lead to a dysfunctional relationship. This may often be the case with safeguarding issues, where the health worker might have to accept unpleasant facts about the parental attitude towards their infant. This will not only compromise their own approach but pose the decision whether to refer onto another agency, considering the factor of paramountcity and the welfare of the child.

Rogers developed 'unconditional positive regard', a concept which encouraged the therapist to accept and not judge the client. This raises the question about the health worker's own attitudes and values. This can be particularly important when listening to the reasons why a parent has contemplated suicide and expresses those negative thoughts. Rogers found that the ability of the listener to convey a non-judgemental attitude provided the positive conditions which enabled the person's personal growth and helped them to understand why negative thoughts have been overwhelming.

It has been found that the more confident the person, the more they are able to listen (Clark 1989). However, those who are less confident about talking appear to be more capable of being receptive for the emotional meaning when they listen. The ability to listen is positively correlated with communication skills (Roberts & Vinson 1998). When speaking, over half of the meaning is translated non-verbally, while Mehrabian (1981) found that under 10 per cent is actually communicated by words alone.

The average rate of speech is approximately 120–180 words per minute, but the health worker should be able to listen to around 450 words per minute (Carver *et al.* 1970). Barker and Watson (2000) suggested that listening is done through one of four primary styles which include the orientation to people, time, action and content, with half of individuals choosing to listen with one or two distinct styles. Whether gender is an issue in the way listening occurs is debatable, but females are found to be more people orientated, while males tend toward action and time.

The most helpful listening skills are the ability to provide the space to allow emotions to be fully expressed and just 'to be there' as a support, which is often a pre-requisite for a health worker. Active listening has been shown to have increased compliance and the perception of a supportive atmosphere (Hausman 2001, Wanzer *et al.* 2004).

It is therefore important to explore the skills of the listener and attend to the basic rules of engagement, the actual environment and the perceived outcomes.

Here is a checklist to think about before entering into conversation with the mother:

1 Which room do I use?
2 What about the baby?
3 Where do I sit?
4 Assuming the counselling pose
5 How long do I spend there?

1 Explore the suitability of the room

A kitchen or patio area may be preferable to other over-crowded living areas, where distractions of the television, computers, iphones and telephones may be a problem. However, if there is no choice about the environment, then consideration should be given to the options. This is where 'ground rules' are useful as part of the contract between you and the mother. There is no need to formalise it, but use as a part of the opening expectations. It could be suggested that interruptions are minimised, for example: switching off the mobile telephone, not answering the landline, turning the television off or onto mute, avoiding answering the door, dissuading friends etc from visiting, postponing callers. Minimise or stop outside noises by asking that washing machines, spin driers, music stations, including your own mobile phone, are switched off. The time you will be spending will be limited and therefore predicting all the eventualities which may disturb or disrupt your session is vital.

2 What about the baby?

The inevitable question is asked about the baby – should the baby be present? There are mixed reviews, but it is sometimes understood that during difficult moments, the mother may find something to divert her thought processes, and attention to the infant is probably the most effective and the most difficult to stop. This is the mother's time and although your focus is on her and her infant, in some research, findings have suggested that the health worker has appeared to be more concerned with the well-being of the infant and less with that of the mother. Allowing the focus to be on the infant can detract from the mother's therapy. Ideally the infant could be cared for during the session and be returned at the end of the listening session.

3 Where do I sit?

This might be obvious to the experienced health worker, but to the novice or inexperienced health worker may cause anxiety, as quick judgements have to be made about the correct seating position. In an office or counselling room, preparations can be made before-hand, but moving furniture and altering spaces in another person's home may be intrusive. It is important to remember spacing and intimate spaces. How close is too close? Ideally sitting close enough is having the ability to reach out and touch, as in comforting, or to hand a tissue, but sitting too far away and feeling the need to jump up to comfort someone is daunting for both. Chairs should ideally be at 45 degrees to each other, enabling eye contact and the ability to read each other's body language. It is probable you may be listening to someone who is suffering from severe anxiety so the pitch and volume of a voice can help them to relax. Soft, modulated tones convey warmth, whereas loud and aggressive tones can cause and promote anxiety and unease, while stilted or stoic speech can be distractive (Edwards & Darley 2002, Engleberg 2006).

4 Body language

Non-verbal communication in the form of body language is important; it can be taken for granted that every health worker is aware of the correct pose to assume when listening. Relaxed shoulders, open arms, legs splayed, head to one side, eyes making contact. These convey all the signs that you are calm, receptive and ready to listen. In reality this is far more difficult to achieve. While you are checking your position is receptive, this in itself may be disturbing for the mother. Remember to be relaxed, you may hear something exhilarating, exciting or inventive, or you may feel as if you have heard it all before. Whatever you hear, you have to hear it and while you concentrate on how you appear, you might miss something vital. Perhaps one of the easiest ways to 'check' that you have achieved the listening pose is to look at the mother's position. Is her stance mirroring yours? Is her hand supporting her chin or folded in her lap? What about yours? Are her legs crossed? What about yours? The chances are that if you are really listening, your body language will mirror hers.

5 How long do I spend there?

Health workers may be confused about the amount of time you should spend listening, and have suggested that it can range from fifteen minutes to two hours. Research into time limits on listening explains that it depends on the preparation and interest of the listener. For example the maximum time for students to absorb information in a lecture is fifteen minutes and after twenty minutes they cease listening (Tough 2012). There is little need to exhaust either the mother or yourself. The suggested listening time is an hour, with plans to conclude the listening time in fifty minutes. This allows the mother to know a start and stop time. 'I will be here at 10 am and will leave at 11 am'. (This would be expected from any professional or deliveryman. . . . The plumber/parcel will be there between 1 and 3 pm). Ensure that a clock or watch is clearly visible to enable you to monitor the time, without looking awkwardly at your watch or the clock in the corner.

The preparations are:

- arrive at the appointed time
- check the room/environment is suitable
- note where you will be sitting
- switch off all electronic devices
- check your pose
- check the time
- have tissues ready

WHY LISTENING IS IMPORTANT

Listening is important because it is not merely hearing what is being said, but how it is being said, what inferences are made and what is unspoken. It is only when the complexities of this process are mastered that it could be possible to create a computer software program to replace the role of health workers, but until that time we have to rely on individuals to be effective listeners.

It is a basic human need to want to be heard. We would all admit to needing to be listened to at some point and everyone has experienced the frustration of not having their point of view heard or even ignored. As children we learnt the importance of listening; and the adage that 'children should be seen and not heard' has long been vanquished to allow children, too, to voice their concern to be listened to.

Perinatal mental health issues are important and need to be listened to. Studies have frequently quoted parents who feel that professionals have demonstrated little regard for their well-being and placed more emphasis on the care of their infant. They object to not feeling listened to, and in the morass of their busy lives, while coping with their new role of motherhood as well as their old roles, the need for added attention can easily be missed. Parents sometimes feel the need to be instructed or told what to do but often it is in the parent's best interest to be helped to reach a solution to the problem.

Employing this philosophy can be a daunting task for some health workers as it contravenes the need for prescriptive interventions. Health workers, as facilitators, operate primarily to resolve or repair problems and often there is a tendency to offer solutions. However, the key to the listening visit is empathetic responses, to expand the skills of listening by paraphrasing, reflecting and summarising what the parent has said. The clear understanding of the difference between thoughts and feelings can clarify the parent's reasoning. The explanation of the parent's emotions, experiences and consequent behaviours can transport thoughts from a superficial to a more intense level. The parent's core beliefs are underlying schemas held about themselves, others and the environment and are usually derived from early experiences. Maintaining this attention to detail allows the mother to remain focused and, as a partnership, the mother and health worker can explore coping strategies, problem solving and cognitive behavioural techniques.

Everyone wants consideration of and agreement with their view point and we demand that what we express is validated and respected, even if our thoughts are sometimes erroneous. Listening without thinking is a specific requirement for respecting the other's position. This will be difficult if the attention is primarily on yourself and you are preoccupied with your own thoughts. The ability to develop this skill is demanding, as we often listen for the weakness or controversial statement as well as the enlightened or liberal ones which may or may not be in agreement with our own opinions. We might consider how we will respond to those comments or even try to justify how we would feel in a similar situation. It is a demanding task to stop your intrusive thoughts but you can learn to ignore them and focus on what is being said. Should the parent feel their opinion is not respected they will suspect you do not understand their situation and consider you a poor listener.

EMPATHETIC RESPONSES

As part of our emotional make-up we have the ability to share and understand the experiences of others and the feelings they may encounter. Imagine you have just stubbed your toe or jammed your fingers in the door. It hurts, you can feel the pain and you wince. When someone talks about that sort of pain you are able to imagine it and not have to physically perform the act to empathise with it. Equally you may empathise with the grief and loss someone is experiencing, but may find it difficult to empathise with the mother who was depressed and starved her infant or the father who lost control and hit his child.

Health workers may spend many hours training to perfect their existing skills by practising the art of listening intently. In order to listen well it is important to put thoughts aside and try to experience what the other person is feeling. Be attentive to the words they are expressing and the deep emotions which may accompany them. One expression is 'putting yourself in their shoes' or 'having a fellow feeling in one's bosom'. It requires you to develop the relationship with the parent, that allows them to feel sufficiently relaxed to enable them to talk unreservedly. You have the privilege of entering their private world and feeling at home.

Empathy can be low or even absent in the parent who faces the challenge of depression. Similarly it is difficult for the parent who is suffering from a psychotic episode and finds it difficult to face reality. It is important to recognise and not to react to the depth of a parent's despair, not to become entangled in the negative reactions 'I just cannot see the point of anything, this is so tedious, you look bored, you really are wasting your time with me, you should go', but to listen to what is really being said. It is probable that parents with depressive symptoms will have negative thoughts and feelings which permeate throughout the dialogue. It is sometimes difficult not to collude with those feelings and be aware of an element of sympathy, to agree with the negative attitude. However, using positive regard it is more important to challenge this negativity with a sensitive, positive attitude to help them to focus on their inner strengths: that they are a good parent, and possess favourable attributes which can override any negative statements (Howe 2012).

It is the ability to keep an open mind to allow yourself to discover the merit or value of what is being said. An extraordinary feeling is not knowing why you understand the inner strength or self-worth of the parent, or that something that is said seems to makes perfect sense. This sentiment may be couched in the terms of intuition or instinct, but it is about recognising your own wisdom, which is brought about by the thirst for knowledge about people and the innumerable ways in which they behave and react. When you consistently believe in people's positive qualities and potential, your own potential is reinforced.

INITIATING THE PROCESS

The use of open questioning will help to generate the conversation and allow problems to be examined in more depth. This is a question which cannot be answered with a 'yes' or 'no' but allows a more free-flowing conversation. As an example, 'How are you feeling today?' will receive a more open response than 'Are you feeling okay today?' (Nelson-Jones 1988, Egan 1986).

REFLECTION

Reflection is the process of reflecting back what you have heard to indicate that you have understood what has been said, sometimes referred to as 'checking'. This assures the parent they have been listened to and understood and if there are any misunderstandings or misconceptions, this provides the opportunity to correct them. It will also make them more aware of their feelings. This enables the listener to confirm and consolidate what has been heard and to construct a framework which allows further exploration of the issues.

PARAPHRASING

Paraphrasing permits the listener to clarify what has been heard and by considering the meaning, helps the parent hear what they have just said. For example:

Mother: 'I was so energetic, I could work all day and then get on with the housework when I got home. These days I can't find the time to do anything except feed the baby, not that I object to that, it is just I seem to be running around in circles with nothing to show for it.'

Listener rephrasing: 'You feel you're using so much energy with nothing to show for it?

Listener paraphrasing: 'You were energetic and had managed your busy lifestyle. However at the moment you feel there is little time for anything except feeding the baby. You don't object to that but you feel for all your efforts you have nothing to show for it. Have I understood that correctly?

REFLECTING FEELINGS

As well as reflecting back thoughts it is also important to reflect feelings. In the example below the feelings are in italics.

I am so *angry*. I was always the best at my work, getting things done on time, managing clients, getting the reports finished. Now I am *so tired* and *so stupid*, I can't seem to *get anything done*. I am *such a mess*.

The words have been changed to reflect what the listener has heard.

Angry = out of control
Tired = lethargic
Stupid = slow
Get anything done = unable to manage
Such a mess = muddled

'You were able to manage but now you feel as if your life is out of control. You feel lethargic and this makes you slow. You feel muddled and unable to cope with your lifestyle. Have I understood this correctly?' Thus offering the mother the opportunity to listen to your interpretation and agree or correct any assumptions (Marcé Resource Pack 2012).

SUMMARISING

At the end of the listening session it is helpful if you briefly summarise what has been said.

For example:

> Let me try to recap what you've told me today. You feel angry that you do not have any time for yourself, and you feel your mother should be able to help more. You have refused her help so far but you think she would be happy to take the baby for a few hours each day. You will have a chat to her about how you feel and will arrange for her to have the baby on Tuesday.

COMPLEX APPROACHES

Active listening ensures that all the information you receive is registered, but another skill is being aware of what is not spoken or said – the hidden clues. You may have developed a trusting relationship and established a sound rapport, but there is a doubt that the parent has not fully revealed how they truly feel either because they are embarrassed or want to avoid confrontation. As communication is on various levels, often they may believe they are divulging secrets or their discomfort that you fail to interpret or acknowledge. For example she may say 'I am such a bad parent'. There is a temptation to react by being judgemental and suggest she is not, but this does not allow her to understand why she feels bad, so reiterating the word 'bad?', will encourage further exploration of what she means by that. Being able to recognise the hidden meaning in the narrative takes skill and patience. One skill is to decipher the level of commitment, sincerity and integrity to be able to understand why they would behave in this way, but also to acknowledge if it requires effort to ignore issues that might be confrontational or cause discomfort.

ANGER

The expression of anger or annoyance is not always apparent, but may be perceptible. It is sometimes difficult to be attentive if the content of the mother's dialogue is threatening, but one of the prerequisite listening skills is to be non-judgemental, and it is important not to be defensive or react when confronted by an angry parent. They may not be aware of their anger but equally may feel threatened and therefore the response is automatic. It is important that the anger is reflected and deflected. Body language is important as any defensive reaction might be interpreted as aggression, therefore remaining relaxed and calm will help to diffuse the situation.

For example:

> *Parent*: 'I am sick and tired of you sitting there saying nothing constructive. We are trying our best but you don't seem to understand that we need help.'
>
> *Listener*: 'You feel I am not helping because I am not telling you what to do?'
>
> *Parent*: 'That's right . . . no, I mean I just want you to say something to help me out here?'
>
> *Listener*: 'You want me to say something to help?'
>
> *Parent*: 'Yes, like how I can manage my day by sorting out my life. Like – could my mother help to look after the baby or what friends do I have. . . .'

TEARS AND JOY

Crying in public is not always socially acceptable and it may prove uncomfortable for both the parent and the listener. The parent may feel stupid and ashamed, but equally may need to release the intensity of the emotion. The listener may feel embarrassed and not know whether to stop the crying or allow it to happen naturally. The decision is dependent on the situation and an understanding of the emotional content of the session. Remaining calm and silent, and offering tissues can help the parent to resolve her emotions quietly and with dignity (Aldridge 2014).

Equally the situation might arise when the sentiment of the parent's 'story' may provoke emotions within the listener and may raise the question of whether it is appropriate to react. As the process of listening is a deeply human one, and when the right conditions prevail, a demonstration of empathy by a tear or sniff, are probably more assuring to the parent than a nod or sound. The detail is in the intensity of the emotion. The tears of the listener are less therapeutic than the tears of the parent.

Humour and joy are also acceptable. Expressions of empathy that mirror the parent's delight or enchantment can help in the recovery process. To share a joke or laugh, with the parent, at an absurd situation, is natural and often stimulating. For the parent whose enjoyment of life is stilted, one such moment can make a significant impact on both the sentiment of the therapeutic approach and the demeanour of the session (Bennett & Lengacher 2008).

SILENCES

Sometimes silent periods within a visit may make health workers feel uncomfortable or awkward and you would rather talk to fill the space. Often the parent may not be aware of the silence as they may be collecting their thoughts or taking the time to think about what has just been said. Passively sitting holding your own thoughts is a powerful moment of acceptance.

PATIENCE

Trust takes a long time to establish and one of the qualities of a listener is having the ability to be patient. This may be frustrating as you may feel your time has been exploited or that you are repeatedly returning to the same topic area and covering identical issues. It may be difficult not to prejudge the value of what is being said because you may have had similar experiences with many other parents and have preconceived notions about the format of the conversation which is unlikely to contain anything worthwhile. It is easy to pretend to listen while not paying any attention. This might be the case but, equally, parents will often claim they had to constantly reiterate the same thoughts and feelings to enable them to understand or make sense of them. Some have been unaware of this repeated exercise but others, who are 'stuck', may need gentle persuasion or alternative avenues to help them move on.

For example, asking the questions:

'What made your day better yesterday?'

'What made your day worse?'

Or

'Who did you find the most helpful?'

'Who did you find the least helpful?'

Or

'How do you think your behaviour will affect your child in 20 years' time?'

Problem solving exercises might help the parent who finds it difficult to move forward, using cognitive behavioural therapy techniques.

For depressed parents, their speech may be slow, monotonous and monosyllabic at times which can prove frustrating for both parties. One prerequisite is patience, to allow the time for the parent to gather their thoughts. One of the many symptoms will be lack of concentration, which will make rapid or even sensible responses, difficult. Responses may be delayed and there may be times when long periods of silence are born out of the inability to express thoughts, rather than not knowing the answer or telling the story. They may be only too aware of the silences and experience discomfort, if they know you are waiting for the response. Careful assurance that you are not in any rush or that it is quite acceptable to take their time can help to pacify them. If the conversation becomes stilted, it might be acceptable to discontinue the session, and suggest that they try to either write down what they were trying to articulate or record their thoughts onto a voice recorder, to enable you to discuss it on your next visit. A wise woman once said 'Before you can reassure someone you have to assure them first'.

SUICIDE AND INFANTICIDE

Contrary to popular opinion, pregnancy and motherhood do not protect mothers against having suicidal thoughts or committing suicide. The last three Confidential Enquiries into Saving Mothers' Lives (2006–2008) found that maternal suicide was more common than previously thought and was a leading overall cause of maternal death, although suicide during pregnancy remained relatively uncommon. The suicide rate was substantially elevated in women who suffered from a severe mental illness. The demographic evidence suggests that over half of the maternal suicides were Caucasian, married, employed, living in comfortable circumstances and aged 30 years or older. In contrast, suicides associated with substance misuse were mostly young women who were single and unemployed.

It may be thought as a privilege to share the thoughts of someone who is feeling vulnerable and who has contemplated suicide, but equally it brings into sharp focus our own thoughts of why a mother or father would kill either themselves or their defenceless child. Emotive words may be conjured up by the media who describe parents as 'crazy', 'mad' or 'disturbingly dangerous' and it may be uncomfortable to acknowledge that rather than 'bad' the parents are 'mad' for denying their child the right to a parent or a child to a life.

Some suggest that the safety of the location and the mindset of the parent to allow us to hear them, are important. The reasons for contemplating suicide are often multi-factorial, but sometimes just a state of mind. A clear understanding of the severity of the symptoms of anxiety and depression can justify why parents would want to end their lives or that of their child. They are often unable to comprehend the damage they may inflict, but quite conversely, are convinced about the lack of pressures and benefits for others. In Malaysia, Razali *et al.* (2014) examined the background of mothers who were found guilty of filicide (the act of a parent killing their child) and found that the mothers were disaffected and had complex social and psychological needs. They presented with maladaptive ways in which to cope with their life stressors, which included self-harm and anger. It was suggested the mothers faced potentially unjust prison sentences for filicide.

CONFIDENTIALITY

The British Association of Counselling and psychotherapy (www.bacp.vo.uk) has an ethical framework for respecting privacy and confidentiality which advises that 'Respecting clients' privacy and confidentiality are fundamental requirements for keeping trust and respecting client autonomy'. It suggests that information may be disclosed if it is authorised by the client or by the law. In exceptional circumstances it may be difficult to seek the consent to the client because they may be causing serious harm to themselves or others. This would be the case in safeguarding cases. However, to ensure that trust and confidence in the listening process is not broken, it is always preferable to seek the consent of the parent before referring to social services or to other statutory organisations. Mitchels and Bond (2010) recommend that listeners have a sound knowledge about the law requirements and confidentiality.

KEEPING A DIARY

The parent could be requested to complete a Mood / Food / Booze / Snooze Diary between the Listening visits. This would enable the parent to record moods, diet, alcohol and sleep patterns, which may a prove a valuable asset.

EXERCISE 4.1

What are your thoughts when you read the following?

Mrs A, aged 36 years, a wealthy gold merchant, was found hanged in her luxury penthouse. Her 3-month-old daughter was out with the nanny at the time.

Ms B, a 26-year-old drug user, was found dead from an overdose of heroine. Her 6-week-old son was found asleep at her side.

The body of Mr C, a 32-year-old social worker, was found by his 4-year-old son, in the seat of his fume-filled car. His partner and his 5-week-old twin boys were in hospital at the time.

It is worth checking your thoughts on this

What are your initial thoughts?

- Who is to blame?
- Why did they do it?
- What factors drove them to do this?
- With the complex knowledge and skills you will have acquired about parental mental illness you will understand the hopelessness and helplessness that some parents feel and how they might have suicidal ideation.

This is what might have happened if they had been asked how they are feeling:

Mrs A, a wealthy gold merchant, told you she has had thoughts of ending it all by hanging herself from the banister on the landing. She has felt depressed for a very long time – she can't remember how long, but she does not feel she can go on like this. She has made plans for weeks now but the time never seems right. She was going to do it on the day the nanny insisted on taking her daughter for a walk to the park, which is several miles away. Mrs A says she has always felt a successful business woman but a useless mother and is a poor substitute for the nanny who always seems to make her daughter smile and giggle. Her daughter always cries when

Mrs A holds her, and she seems to prefer the nanny. It makes perfect sense to not inflict herself on her daughter any further and if she were out of the picture it would mean the nanny would take good care of her daughter and it would free up her husband to find someone else. You are the first person who has asked her if she has had thoughts of harming herself and she suddenly feels relieved (and stupid) talking about how she really feels for the first time.

Ms B said sometimes she felt like ending it all. She hated not being able to give up the feeling the drugs gave her, which was hope. When she was high she really felt she could manage her son. She said that sometimes when she was at her lowest, she just wanted to feel high all the time. She never had any real plans, but the thought of eternal peace was sometimes overwhelming and just one more hit would have made it 'right' this time. Everyone judged her all the time and the social services did not seem to give her a chance. Perhaps if she did end it all her son would be adopted by better parents, who did not rely on drugs. She is glad you asked and did not dismiss her actions but allowed her to talk freely about what she felt, without being judged.

Mr C had been informed several months ago they were going to make cuts to social services and that his position was untenable. He had to consider the possibility of moving to another area to secure a better job. He was already on the lowest pay scale and finding it increasingly difficult to manage the mortgage on his wages. When his wife announced she was pregnant with twins, he did not know how they would continue to pay the bills. His wife had brought in a second income but now the prospect of her having to give up work was overwhelming. She had a history of depression and had been admitted to the local psychiatric hospital with a psychotic episode. The twins were being cared for by a cousin in another part of town. He tried to think of options but his head 'was all over the place'. Mr C could not bear the thought of being such a failure, unable to support his family who would probably be better off without him. He is embarrassed that you asked, but talking about it has made him realise that although there are an enormous amount of problems, there are also solutions, he just needs to ask for help.

Skype and listening

If resources, either financial or personnel, cannot allow the benefit of a listening visit, then other means should be considered. The rapid advances in technology provide the opportunities and challenges for health workers. There is the expectation to keep pace with young clients' needs and priorities. Internet technology is slowly expanding and becoming increasingly popular within the field of health. Most homes have access to a computer or other forms of the internet, making the process of being able to Skype feasible, although technology is notoriously unreliable in some areas. There is the convenience of timing and location. It allows all of the necessary prerequisites – the images of non-verbal as well as verbal communication. Skype can provide therapists with a variety of options for distal contact with their clients that can include visual imagery. This technology opens up new possibilities for exposure treatment for anxiety and behavioural activation for depression, in which the client and therapist may interact in the virtual world together, or the client can interact virtually with social groups (Newman et al. 2011).

Findings by Callahan and Inckle (2012) suggest that the online therapeutic conversations with young people dealt with more sensitive and a greater variety of topics than face-to-face sessions. They also concluded that young people might feel less intimidated talking to an online counsellor and more able to exercise their own power in this context.

Telephone counselling

The Samaritans have used telephone listening for many years and the success rate and continued operation of the organisation are testimony to the efficacy of the programme (www.samaritans.org). It is the point of contact for individuals who have suicidal ideation, need someone to talk with privately and prefer the anonymity of the telephone call.

Minimal contact interpersonal therapies have been proposed as an effective and low cost intervention for parents with anxiety and depressive disorders. Although not ideal, it is possible that this form of listening might be considered for those parents who live in inaccessible areas. Dennis (2014) developed and implemented a telephone-based peer support programme for mothers with postnatal depression. Mothers felt it was convenient and met their treatment needs. The results suggested this may be an effective intervention that reduces the risk of the symptoms at twelve weeks following the birth. A similar scheme in America produced comparable results, providing a safe, efficacious method to reduce symptoms of postnatal depression, reduce fragmented care and provide care for mothers who might otherwise not receive treatment (Posmontier 2014).

In another American study, midwives were trained to administer interpersonal psychotherapy by telephone to women with postnatal depression. This was an expressed requirement as many of the women had complex needs which included poor access to mental health services, competing childcare responsibilities, and resistance to retelling their stories to others. It was found that this type of intervention was well accepted and viewed as feasible and acceptable but more importantly improved the mothers' depressive symptoms.

There are specific courses on telephone counselling but as a rule of thumb the most important requirement is to sound human, caring and real.

As an example:

> *Listener:* Picks up the phone, says 'hello' but there is silence.
> 'It's okay – you can talk whenever you are ready' 'I am here to help'.
> There is a response.
> *Listener:* 'What's your name?'
> *Mother:* 'Sandy Watkins.'
> *Listener:* 'Do you mind if I call you Sandy?'
> *Mother:* 'I have so many problems I don't know where to begin. I feel so alone and so frightened to tell anyone how I feel.'
> *Listener:* 'You have a lot of problems, feel lonely and are frightened to let anyone know – have I got that right?'

Child is crying in the background/dog is barking/television is loud.
Listener acknowledges what she hears.
'Is that a little one I can hear crying?' 'What's her name?' 'Oh that's a pretty
name . . . I have a cousin with that name . . .'

The main points to remember are:

- Make sure you are in a place without background noise to enable you to both hear each other.
- Always ask the parent if this is the telephone I can get you back on if I lose signal.
- Never divulge your personal mobile number, as you might receive a distressed text and are unable to do anything about it.
- Ensure the parent is safe.
- Talk with confidence.
- Always have an opening line, which you have rehearsed.
- Have a beginning, endeavour to have some solution to the parent's problem and an end – what will be the future developments/solutions?
- Let the parent talk, but take control if you find her going off track in your conversation.
- Do not be afraid to ask her to repeat herself if you did not understand what was said.
- Never promise them anything you cannot deliver.
- If the parent feels you are not listening that might jeopardise the rapport.
- Ensure that you will help them get to the right source of help.
- Ensure the last few minutes are the most important part of the call.

When talking over the phone try to visualise the parent in front of you. Sometimes parents feel less confident talking to someone over the phone or you may feel uncomfortable. An opening line, which is familiar to you, always helps you to feel more confident. When I do talks I often use the same paragraph and that triggers my confidence to carry on. Most importantly do not sound like a robot, just be yourself and care (Williams 2014).

Texting

Mobile phone texting allows the opportunity to engage with parents using a medium which is both familiar and accessible. Cartwright and Gibson (2014) studied mobile phone text counselling and found the methods successful. There is however, the difficulty of conveying emotional discourse and there is the danger that without attention to accuracy of the grammar, sentence construction, punctuation and use of abbreviations, the scripts could be misconstrued or misinterpreted. It is also time consuming to the untrained fingers and any delay in the replies may cause undue anxiety to both parties.

EXERCISE 4.2

Punctuation mistakes in texting

Write a text with no punctuation, then write one with the correct punctuation. Demonstrate how it might be misinterpreted.

For example:

> Hi mary i want someone to know what listening is all about you are patient kind and thoughtful health workers who are not like you admit to being incapable of listening and caring i have no one to trust when i know you do not have the time to text me

> Hi Mary, I want someone to know what listening is all about. You are patient, kind and thoughtful. Health workers who are not like you admit to being incapable of listening and caring. I have no one to trust when I know you do not have the time to text me.

> Hi mary i want someone to know what listening is. all about you are patient, kind and thoughtful. health workers who are not like you. admit to being incapable of listening and caring. i have no one to trust. when i know you, do not have the time to text me.

Whatever the method used, the prerequisites are: the skills of being able to understand the background of why parents may not be able to function as they might normally do; to have an awareness of the life changes that perinatal mental illness may bring to a relationship, not only between adults, but of the impact it has on children; and to listen intently, actively, non-judgementally and most importantly with a genuine regard for the parent.

EXERCISE 4.3

Positioning for the listening visit

In pairs – one is **A** and the other is **B**

Where to sit?

This is a simple exercise to establish the best position for listening.

Take two chairs and place them where you think is the ideal site. Sit in the chairs and check position.

Are you:

- Able to lean forward without invading each other's body space?
- Close enough to place your hand on a knee or pass over a handkerchief?
- Comfortable with your position?

When you have established the most comfortable position for you both, take some time to look at each other. This should last for a minute.

A: Stare at **B**'s forehead

Feedback what this feels like, does it make you feel uncomfortable and why?

B: Stare at **A**

A: Look at **B's** chin

B: Look into the distance

Feedback what this feels like, does it make you feel uncomfortable and why?

Often when the talker is recollecting a subject, their eyes might not always be on the Listener and may not maintain eye contact. However, the Listener's eyes should always make contact with the Talker, as when the Talker looks at the Listener, eye contact should be made.

As an example, think about when you are talking to someone. Do you look at them all the time, yet you would expect them to be looking at you?

EXERCISE 4.4

This exercise is designed to help you focus on listening and concentrating – both as a listener and parent

Oral description of object

In pairs – one is **A** and the other is **B**

Both have a piece of paper to draw on and pen.

Sit in chairs which are back to back, so neither can see the other, but ensure that background noise is minimal to ensure you are able to hear

- **A:** thinks of a simple object – for example – an umbrella/a radio/a cat/a pear.
- The shape of the object is described to **B**.
  [Clues are not allowed – for example – 'it is an . . . animal or . . . fruit'. To avoid the use of hand or any other gestures it might be easier to sit on the hands!] This can be done by saying, 'draw a line from the bottom right hand corner to the top of the page'.
- **B:** Draws what is heard and shares the completed drawing with **A.**
- Then to complete the exercise . . .
- **B:** Thinks of a more complex object – for example, a horse and carriage/suit of armour/a crocodile – and repeats the exercise.

This exercise uses only words, or verbal communication, and demonstrates the importance of clear communication with the use of the tone of your voice, pace of speech and intonation. It also demonstrates how important it is for the one who is drawing the object to listen carefully to ensure they clearly understand the instructions.

Examples of where this is important are during counselling using the telephone or when trying to communicate with someone with whom you do not share a common language.

EXERCISE 4.5

This exercise is to focus on the way in which the individual talks and how to take notice of how things are said as well as what is being said

Observing and listening

In a group of two – sitting in the 'Listening' position

One is the Listener and the other is the Talker

- **Talker (Parent):** Think about the three most important things you have in your house and explain why they are significant to you.
- **Listener (Health worker):** Allow the mother to talk uninterrupted – but make note of the facial expressions, body language and tone of voice. Think about her emotions. [Does she sound content, angry, disappointed, distressed?]
- Feedback what the mother has said to you, using your interpretation of her emotions.

For example:

- **You might say:** When you discussed the vase that your aunt had given to you, I noticed you glanced away from me, began twisting your wedding ring and you sounded upset, am I right?
- **Talker:** Yes, I did feel a little tearful when I spoke about it. When you first asked me to name some objects I couldn't think of anything in particular, but then the thought of the vase came into my head and I just realised how important it is to me. I was very close to my aunt and she gave me the vase as a wedding present. My aunt emigrated to Canada shortly afterwards and I miss her.

Allowing the Talker to talk at her own pace while you listen and observe her allows you to generate more 'material' to generate further dialogue.

EXERCISE 4.6

This exercise is designed to help you to understand the barriers which can be created to stop people talking – or listening

During this exercise, A is the parent and B is the health worker. B is told prior to exercise how they are expected to behave. A is unaware of B's intentions

The disrupting visit: 1

In pairs – one is **A** and the other is **B**

- **A (Parent):** speaks for three minutes about *The best part of a Saturday and why*.
- **B (Health worker):** Starts fidgeting in the chair, adjusting clothing, pulling at jumper and scratching the arms.
- **B** feeds back to **A** what this behaviour has meant to the flow of the conversation.

   This exaggerated exercise demonstrates how easy it is for the Listener to be distracted – often subconsciously – and how this affects the ability of **B** to concentrate on their story. They may often say they do not feel 'listened to'.
   This may happen innocently in practice as the Talker may feel strongly that the Listener is eager to get away or feels uncomfortable listening to them. One commented 'She kept jangling her car keys, so I felt she was in a rush to go'.

EXERCISE 4.7

During this exercise, A is the parent and B is the health worker. B is told prior to exercise how they are expected to behave. A is unaware of B's intentions

The disrupting visit: 2

In pairs – one is **A** and the other is **B**

- **A (Parent):** Speaks for three minutes about *The best part of a Saturday and why*.
- **B (Health worker):** Argues with what is being said – for example – 'Oh you may think that is the best part but actually I can't agree with that' or 'If you want my opinion, what you have suggested is probably not the best part at all', or 'I find that suggestion a bit silly'.
- **B** feeds back to **A** what this behaviour has meant to the flow of the conversation.

   These responses are exaggerated and demonstrate how easy it is for the Listener to bring their own beliefs to a visit – and how this affects the ability of **B** to concentrate on their story, because they may feel that what they have to say is unimportant or wrong. They may often say they do not feel 'listened to'.

This may happen innocently in practice as the Listener may feel strongly about a childcare issue – for example, the mother may say she is a vegan and does not want her baby to have cow's milk or the mother feels her baby is too active during the day and wants something to make the baby sleep.

EXERCISE 4.8

During this exercise, A is the parent and B is the health worker. B is told prior to exercise how they are expected to behave. A is unaware of B's intentions

The disrupting visit: 3

In pairs – one is **A** and the other is **B**

- **A (Parent):** Speaks for three minutes about *The best part of a Saturday and why.*
- **B (Health worker):** Agree with what is being said – for example 'Oh you are so right, I love that part of the day too' or 'That is such a good time of the day, you are so smart to get that right' or 'Yes, I completely agree, a great time of day, clever you'.
- **B** feeds back to **A** what this behaviour has meant to the flow of their conversation.

These responses are exaggerated and demonstrate how easy it is for the Listener's listening to be diverted to other situations and how this affects the ability of B to concentrate on their story because they feel patronised and what they say is unimportant. They may often say they do not feel 'listened to'.

This may happen innocently in practice as the Listener may feel strongly that they need to encourage the mother's efforts to make her feel she is doing a good job . . . even though they may not.

EXERCISE 4.9

During this exercise, A is the parent and B is the health worker. B is told prior to exercise how they are expected to behave. A is unaware of B's intentions

The disrupting visit: 4

In pairs – one is **A** and the other is **B**

- **A (Parent):** Speaks for three minutes about *The best part of a Saturday and why.*
- **B (Health worker):** Do not listen to what is being said, but think about what you would do if you won £1 million pounds, had the opportunity to present a television show or were invited to the Palace Garden Party.

■ **B** feeds back to **A** what this behaviour has meant to the flow of their conversation.

These responses are exaggerated and demonstrate how easy it is for the Listener to be preoccupied when something more important happens in their life – and how this affects the ability of the Talker to concentrate on their story because they can sense they are not in the 'bubble' and what they say is unimportant. They may often say they do not feel 'listened to'.

EXERCISE 4.10

During this exercise, A is the parent and B is the health worker. B is told prior to exercise how they are expected to behave. A is unaware of B's intentions

The disrupting visit: 5

In pairs – one is **A** and the other is **B**

■ **A (Parent):** Speaks for three minutes about *The best part of a Saturday and why.*
■ **B (Health worker):** Listen, indicating that you are by nodding your head and uttering, but remain completely quiet – even when **A** stops talking. Try to stay silent as long as possible before you feel uncomfortable and then try to analyse why you feel uncomfortable.
■ **B** feeds back to **A** what this behaviour has meant to the flow of their conversation, while **A** feeds back their thoughts on remaining silent.

This response is exaggerated and demonstrates how easy it is for the Listener to be preoccupied with silences and not take into account how the Talker may be feeling and how this affects the ability of the Talker to concentrate on their story because they can sense they are not in the 'bubble' and what they say is unimportant. They may often say they do not feel 'listened to'.

EXERCISE 4.11

During this exercise, A is the parent and B is the health worker. B is told prior to exercise how they are expected to behave. A is unaware of B's intentions

The disrupting visit: 6

In pairs – one is **A** and the other is **B**

■ **A (Parent):** Speaks for three minutes about *The best part of a Saturday and why.*

■ **B (Health worker):** Bring out your mobile phone and start texting or open up your laptop and start typing. Continue to do this for the three minutes, but indicate you are listening by nodding your head and uttering.

Both feedback what this experience has meant to you.

■ What did they feel when you brought out the device?
■ Did they feel you listened to them?
■ Would they be happy to let you do that again?

This may be an exaggerated scenario but making notes in a laptop has been suggested by some health authorities.

EXERCISE 4.12

What skills are a prerequisite?

Probably one of the first things to consider is what qualities would you require from someone if you wanted them to listen to you?

1 List the qualities of the person you seek out when you need to talk over something that has upset you.
   For example: patience, kindness, calmness.
2 List the irritating factors of the person you avoid when you need to talk over something that has upset you.
   For example: interruptions, disagreements, commands.
3 Write down which of those qualities and irritating factors apply to you.

You know when you are really listening when:

■ you feel as if you are both cocooned in a bubble;
■ you are unaware of outside noises;
■ your body language mirrors that of the mother's;
■ you are surprised how quickly time has passed.

Making notes

Do not make notes during the visit as not only might this be threatening to the mother but will detract from the session. If you have listened well you will have remembered well and be able to write up any notes following the session. That is of course, if you need to? Some employers may insist on some form of paperwork, but in reality there might be little need to write out copious observations. In some areas laptops have been introduced to be used during visits.

EXERCISE 4.13

During this exercise, A is the parent and B is the health worker. B is told prior to exercise how they are expected to behave. A is unaware of B's intentions

Learning patience: 1

In pairs – one is **A** and the other is **B**

■ **A (Parent):** Think about a task you have been meaning to do but have not got around to because something has prevented it.

For example tidying up the shed, but you are unable to throw anything away/weeding the garden, but you have arthritis in your knees/taking up the hem on a piece of clothing but your sewing skills are poor.

Start to talk about what needs to be done and then take time to contemplate how that will be achieved. Make the silences long. This should take about three minutes.

■ **B (Health worker):** Listen and think about how you feel during the session.

Both feedback what this experience has meant to you.

EXERCISE 4.14

During this exercise, A is the parent and B is the health worker. B is told prior to exercise how they are expected to behave. A is unaware of B's intentions

Learning patience: 2

In pairs – one is **A** and the other is **B**

■ **A (Parent):** Talk for three minutes about the contents of your shopping trolley. Repeat several times what you bought and why. For example: 'Yes I have beans, they are good for you, you know, and carrots which are equally good, but did I tell you I bought beans, they are good for you aren't they?'

■ **B (Health worker):** Listen and think about how you feel during the session.

Both feedback what this experience has meant to you.

REFERENCES

Aldridge, S. (2014). *A short Introduction to Counselling*. London: Sage

Barker, L.L. & Watson, K.W. (2000). *Listen up. How to improve relationships, reduce stress and be more productive by using the power of listening*. New York, NY: St Martin's Press

Bennett, M.P. & Lengacher, C. (2008). Humor and laughter may influence health: III: Laughter and health outcomes. *Evidence-Based Complementary and Alternative Medicine* 5:37–40

British Association of Counselling and Psychotherapy. (www.bacp.co.uk)

Callahan, A. & Inckle, K. (2012). Cybertherapy or psychobabble? A mixed methods study of online emotional support. *British Journal of Guidance & Counselling* 40(3):261–278

Cartwright, C. & Gibson, K. (2014). Young people's experiences of mobile phone text counselling: Balancing connection and control. *Children and Youth Services Review* 96–104.

Carver, R.P., Johnson, R.L. & Friedman, H.L. (1970). Factor analysis of the ability to comprehend time-compressed speech. (Final report for the National Institute for health). Washington DC: American Institute for Research

Centre for Maternal and Child Enquiries (CMACE) (2011). Saving Mothers' Lives: reviewing maternal deaths to make motherhood safer: 2006–08. The Eighth Report on Confidential Enquiries into Maternal Deaths in the United Kingdom. *BJOG* 118 (Suppl. 1):1–203.

Clark, A.J. (1989). Communication confidence and listening competence: An investigation of the relationships of willingness to communicate, communication apprehension, and receiver apprehension to comprehension of content and emotional meaning in spoken messages. *Communication Education* 38(3):237–249

Dennis, C-L. (2014). The process of developing and implementing a telephone-based peer support program for postpartum depression: Results from a randomized controlled trial. *Trials* 15:131

Edwards, C. & Darley, M. (2002). Managing *Communication in Health Care*. Edinburgh: Harcourt Publishers Ltd

Egan, G. (1986). *The Skilled Helper*. Pacific Grove, CA: Brooks/Cole

Engleberg, I.N. (2006). Working in groups: Communication principles and strategies. *My Communication Kit Series*:140–141

Hausman, A. (2001). Taking your medicine: Relational steps to improving patient compliance. *Health Marketing Quarterly* 19:49–71

Howe, D. (2012). *Empathy, What it is and Why it Matters*. Basingstoke: Palgrave Macmillan

Marcé Resource Pack (2012). Available from www.marcesociety.com

Mehrabian, A. (1981). *Silent Messages: Implicit Communication of Emotions and Attitudes*. Belmont, CA: Wadsworth

Mitchels, B. & Bond, T. (2010). *Essential Law for Counsellors and Psychotherapists*. London: Sage

Nelson-Jones, R. (1988). *Practical Counselling and Helping Skills*. London: Cassell

Newman, M.G., Szkodny, L.E., Llera, S.J. & Przeworski, A. (2011). A review of technology-assisted self-help and minimal contact therapies for anxiety and depression: Is human contact necessary for therapeutic efficacy? *Clinical Psychology Review* 31(1):89–103

Posmontier, B. (2014). Multidisciplinary model of nurse midwife administered psychotherapy for postpartum depression. In Abstracts for the International

Marce Society for Perinatal Mental Health Biennial Scientific Conference. *Archives of Women's Mental Health* 18(2) published online April 2015

Razali, S. Kirkman, M., Ahmad, S.H. & Fisher, J. (2014). Infanticide and illegal infant abandonment in Malaysia. *Child Abuse Neglect* Jul 18. doi: 10.1016/j.chiabu.2014.06.008

Roberts, C.V. & Vinson, L. (1998). Relationship among willingness to listen, receiver apprehension, communication apprehension, communication competence, and dogmatism. *International Journal of Listening* 12:40–57.

Rogers, C. (1957). The necessary and sufficient conditions of therapeutic personality change. *Journal of Consulting Psychology* 21(2):95–103

The Samaritans. www.samaritains.org

Tough, P. (2012). *Time Education.* www.ideas.time.com

Wanzer, M.B., Booth-Butterfield, M. & Gruber. M.K. (2004). Perceptions of health care providers' communication: Relationships between patient-centered communication and satisfaction. *Health Communication* 16(3):363–384

Weaver, J.B., Richendoller, N.R. & Kirtley, M.D. (1995). *Individual differences in communication style.* Paper presented at the annual meeting of the Speech Communication Association. San Antonio, TX

Williams, M. (2014). Talking with fathers on the telephone (oral communication)

FATHERS AND PERINATAL MENTAL HEALTH

5

Mark Williams

> *Her*: 'You never listen to me'!
> *Him*: 'Yes I do'
> *Her*: 'No you don't!'
> *Him*: 'Yes I do!'
> *Her*: 'No you don't!'
> *Him*: 'Yes I do!!!'
> *Her*: 'You never listen, so shut up!'

As this is a comparatively new area of research, there is limited data of the effects of paternal depression on the cognitive, motor, and socio-emotional development of infants. Some studies have highlighted the impact it may have and in Hong Kong, Koh (2014) found that the role of the father coupled with traditionalism–modernity could moderate the relationship between marital dissatisfaction and paternal anxiety and depression. Traditional fathers who were dissatisfied with their marriage were more susceptible to paternal anxiety and depression in late pregnancy and at six weeks post postnatally. Studies in rural Vietnam found that although domestic violence is a crime, young women were still subjected to it and, as in the United Kingdom, it is associated with an increased risk of ante- and postnatal common mental health disorders. Fisher *et al.* (2013) and other researchers have advocated that as a result of these findings there should be community-based violence reduction strategies, which would concentrate on awareness and skills to reduce the incidence. This stresses the importance of the ability to access help in order to sustain and maintain good quality relationships throughout the perinatal period.

Managing men's mental health needs is somewhat different from managing those of women, as fathers who are depressed tend to direct their feelings towards anger, conflict and/or hostility. Their overall responsibilities in caring and childcare have often been marginalised by health workers and it is often evident that fathers tend not to seek help, but prefer to avoid contact or withdraw into escapist activities by overworking, indulging in sport, or self-medication, using alcohol or drugs (Veskrna 2010, Hanley 2013). Accepting this reactive behaviour can be difficult; nevertheless, Mark Williams, who has worked with men for several years, offers the following advice:

The importance of good communication skills cannot be overestimated when talking with fathers as men do not tend to be as communicative about distressful events as women. One of the main openings for a conversation is body language with non-verbal cues. The first fifteen seconds may be the difference between creating an instant rapport with the father or creating a barrier. Talking with any father who is struggling to assimilate his thoughts can be difficult and therefore the health worker must have a certain level of knowledge and control. For many fathers it may be the first time that they are able to unload their problems, so it is important that their voice is heard.

ENVIRONMENT

There are several issues to consider before embarking on a listening visit with a father. The venue is important and ideally should be free of noise and distractions. If the room is full of other people, access to a quiet space or room is preferable. If in the family home and family members are anxious to take part in the conversation, ensure people sit in a triangular format to enable everyone to be seen and join in.

PERSONAL SPACE

When first introducing yourself it is essential to be aware of the space between you and the father, as some fathers may be uncomfortable having their space invaded by a stranger. Sitting opposite and at slight angle is normally the easiest way. Awareness of body language and the messages this conveys is significant, for example, folding your arms when talking to the father suggests that you are holding yourself back and being defensive. Avoiding eye contact or making no eye contact can make communication difficult for the father and suggest to him that you are disinterested in what he has to say. This can be evident with technology, as it is easy to be distracted by an iphone or laptop computer. That momentary lapse of concentration and contact can have a significant impact on the father, particularly if he is feeling vulnerable, and any excuse which might indicate you are not listening will persuade him to shut down.

The tone of voice is crucial, both in one-to-one conversations and group discussions and can make a difference to the reaction of the father. Saying 'How are you?' with soft tones can come across differently from saying it in a brusque or harsh voice. When talking to fathers never search for something to say, as this can make the situation uncomfortable.

Talking and using body language are important to allow the father to gain trust. An acknowledgment of how the father is feeling can be as simple as a nod of the head. When talking to fathers it is important that they feel you understand their frustration. This can be as simple as 'I remember a friend going through a similar situation. . . .'

Fathers need to convey how they are feeling, and will appreciate the use of open questioning, starting sentences with 'how?', 'when?', 'why?', 'where?', 'what?' and 'who?' will allow the father to feel he can reply. Non-verbal communication represents two-thirds of communication with fathers. First encounters or interactions with the father strongly affect his perception. When absorbing the message, they are focused on the entire environment using all five senses during the interaction: 83 per cent sight, 11 per cent hearing, 3 per cent smell, 2 per cent touch and 1 per cent taste.

This is useful if there is a silent pause:

- 'What kind of support do you have from your family?' Pause . . . eye contact. . . .
- 'Where is the mother now?' Pause . . . eye contact. . . .
- 'How are you coping with all this?' Pause . . . eye contact. . . .

When talking to fathers, it is important to take into account how they acquire information. When trying to explain certain situations, some fathers would rather see it written down. It is important to ensure that the father has full view of what is being written, to give him the confidence to know that it is being interpreted correctly.

Listening skills are more necessary than talking skills. If a young father is telling you something that has just happened and you start talking over him, that conversation may be the last open and truthful conversation. If he does not think that you are fully listening then you will miss the underlying issues that are causing his distress. The father should feel that he is able to talk freely. One of the hardest things about fathers opening up about perinatal mental illness in the family is often the lack of education about the illness. The mother may ask the father not to discuss their family issues with anyone, to avoid social services being informed.

Studies have shown that it is positive to experience some anxiety, as a part of the body's make-up. It is okay to feel like that and there is little need to worry about feeling that way. Fathers who have never experienced anxiety before cannot understand why they should experience this, as having a newborn baby in the family should ideally be a happy time. There is often the feeling that anxiety is associated with terrible situations, but it is normal for the father to feel a little anxious, as this is something he truly cares about, the baby and the mother.

COPING SKILLS

In some cases, the fathers have developed negative coping skills and feel they are unable to cope. The provision of stories about personal situations can enable fathers to see similarities in their own lives. Many fathers feel isolated and that they are the only ones who have experienced this. They need to understand that other fathers have had similar experiences. Nearly half of the fathers who have been in contact have developed negative coping skills within a few months of the mother developing perinatal mental health problems. It is helpful to provide the father with positive thoughts to which he can relate, for example from past experiences of helping others.

FURTHER VISITS

The essential messages should be at the beginning and the end of the conversation, ensuring the most important parts are at the end. The father is more likely to take in the last five minutes of the conversation than the middle part. The father should be aware that if he does not want to make the next appointment he must phone to cancel, and there should be a time limit for the cancellation period. Ensure they are aware how valuable (and free) the visit is, as often they may feel that it is less importance to cancel because it is free. It is important to consider a follow-up appointment and direct questioning will give you control. For example:

'So John, I can come and meet you on either Thursday or Friday?' . . . Pause . . . Wait until he answers.

GROUPS

When working with groups of fathers, ground rules should be set at the beginning. It is more relaxed sitting in a circle where everyone is able to be seen. The chair of the facilitator (health worker) should be slightly to the front to enable all the fathers to be seen and to assist with communication. Group confidentiality must be ensured before each meeting, as this will provide fathers with the confidence to open up about their true feelings. Protocols should be enforced about the use of social media and the importance of not divulging any information about the group or individual fathers. The group should be made aware of their safety risks as sometimes there may be more underlying issues than just perinatal mental health in the family and it must be reinforced that the support you are giving is only for their mental well-being.

Open discussions can be begun by anyone in the group. Not all fathers in the group will talk openly, so it's good practice to offer one-to-one support either before the next meeting or at the end. Sometimes a father may monopolise the group, talking longer than necessary about his family's problems. Giving the father a pen to hold as an indication that he is the only father who has a right to talk normally stops others talking over and among themselves.

Dress is important. Prior to convening a fathers' support group, consideration should be given to what is worn as this can make an impact. Casual smart appears to be the more acceptable. If the group feels the health worker is inappropriately dressed, this will determine how they will react, which can sometimes be in a negative way.

Fathers like to see their concerns listed on paper and during each group session each concern is discussed within a certain time scale. Coping skills such as mindfulness and cognitive behavioural therapy help them to understand that there is an avenue for extra help.

Group sessions and support for the facilitator

It is useful to bring in another health worker to the group who can also be involved in the duty of care to the fathers. Some fathers have struggled with a lack of support and this can come across in group sessions. Fathers can bring negative issues revolving around coping skills. Fathers can be signposted to the support they need for problems with alcohol or severe social anxiety.

Sub-groups

The fathers are welcome to form sub-groups outside of the main group, while ensuring the strict group rules are applied and enforced. Anecdotal evidence has suggested that men, unlike women, prefer to discuss their more intimate thoughts while they are occupied and situated side by side. For example, two men together digging up the road, or sharing a game of football, where they feel the environment is safe and secure. In recognition of this behaviour, several groups are adapting this idea by forming 'men sheds'. This initiative copies the idea of a shed, but is larger, where men can feel safe and pursue their practical interests. Groups of men are able to share the tools and resources necessary to work on the projects they choose to work on. It provides a friendly, inclusive atmosphere which allows men to talk openly and freely about issues or problems which have been a source of distress (UK Men's Sheds).

TELEPHONE LISTENING

Listening allows fathers to unburden their worries. When talking to fathers over the telephone it is worth ascertaining if it is appropriate to phone them back on the telephone they are currently using.

Talking to fathers over the telephone can be difficult as facial expressions cannot be seen. This is important if something is said which triggers a negative reaction. Ensure a note pad is available to take notes, and make sure the father is aware of what you are doing. Always clarify what has been said as sometimes the father may be worried, anxious or feel low, making him difficult to understand.

If the father is expressing suicidal thoughts, he must be directed to a helpline telephone number and advised that he must phone this at the end of your phone call, and ensure he attends the next support group. Personal mobile phone numbers should never be revealed to either fathers or families, as, for instance, if the father is expressing suicidal ideation and is unable to contact you, he may leave a suicide note as a text.

Creating a rapport with the father enables him to connect with you. Although this is a technological age people still need to connect with people. It should feel as if you are selling him a wonderful service which will get the right results. A confident pace and tone of voice will assure the father you can deliver the right messages and understand the problems he faces.

Ensure the last few phrases of your conversation are assuring.

For example:

■ 'John, I'm going to find out what debt advisors are really helpful in your area.'
■ 'John, I know you're finding it hard to cope at the moment, but I am able to help you to put something in place.'
■ 'John, I'm going to meet up with you next week, what time is best?'
■ 'John, where shall we meet next week?'

EXERCISE 5.1

Ten top tips for fathers

1 Educate yourself about this illness; there are so many sites on perinatal mental health.
2 Talk to family and friends; tell them how you are really feeling. Educate them too.
3 Exercise and eat healthily.
4 Look for support and for other fathers going through this illness . . . Don't isolate yourself.
5 Support you partner and keep assuring her you will both get through this together.
6 Interact with your newborn and children as much as you can . . . both walks and fresh air are good.
7 Look at coping skills like relaxation classes; avoid using alcohol to cope with stress.
8 If you're feeling low make sure your first call is your GP, and seek other advice if your GP does not understand.
9 Remember in the next ten years 1 million families in the UK will experience this illness.
10 Remember this is an illness, like any other illness. Don't suffer in silence.

Top 10 tips for health workers

1 Ask the father how he is coping.
2 Provide the father with information about perinatal mental health.
3 Ask him if there is support from family and friends.
4 Let the father talk, and listen.

5   Empathy and the assurance that many other fathers have the same experience is vital.
6   Due to timescale for health visitors, it is important to have some preparation on coping skills, websites on perinatal mental health and support groups in the area.
7   Never make promises you can't keep; be honest, this will help to develop the rapport.
8   Encourage the family to go for walks and interact with the newborn/children.
9   Ensure the family knows that thousands of families go through this illness and the quicker the help, the quicker the recovery.
10 Make a point that it is important that both parents are included in this care.

REFERENCES

Fisher, J.R., Tran, T.D., Biggs, B., Dang, T.H., Nguyen, T.H. & Tran, T. (2013). Intimate partner violence and perinatal common mental disorders among women in rural Vietnam. *International Health* 5:29–37

Hanley, J. (2013). Fathers and postnatal depression. *Nursing in Practice Health Visitor Supplement*, May/June 5

Koh, Y.W. (2014). The moderating effect of gender role and traditional modernity of the relationship of marital dissatisfaction and paternal anxiety and depression in Hong Kong. In Abstracts for the International Marce Society for Perinatal Mental Health Biennial Scientific Conference. *Archives of Women's Mental Health* 18(2) published online April 2015

UK Men's Sheds Association. www.menssheds.org.uk

Veskrna, L. (2010). Peripartum depression – does it occur in fathers and does it matter? *Journal of Men's Health* 7(4):420–430

LISTENING TO INFANTS

6

INFANTS

The first 3 years of an infant's life are the most important and, during the early months, his mother in particular is the main source of highly arousing, visually affective communication. A myriad of informatics form the immature brain, stimulating both his social and cognitive development.

From the moment of birth infants mutually interact with their parents. They are not passive recipients of care but actively orchestrate their social contact. Developing infants are highly competent communicators and are able, by the primitive sounds of cooing, gurgling or grunting, to attract attention. The expression in the resonance can help to direct the parent towards their joy, contentment, fear or frustration. Despite having the capacity to imitate others' facial movements, newborn infants demonstrate little spontaneous imitation during face-to-face contact, possibly due to their fundamental capacity to link their experience with that of others (Murray 2014).

As they develop, the infant's listening skills are gained from interactions with both adults and other children. There will be the realisation that certain words have particular meaning. At around 9 months the infant begins to vocalise with meaning, with the first real words expressed at between 15 and 18 months. Linkage of words commences around the age of 18 months to 2 and a half years, and with it, the ability to understand commands. At 3 years they should be able to carry out three commands with ease – for example 'Please go into the kitchen and bring me a bowl from the counter and a spoon from the table'.

The use of making eye contact and facial expressions will help infants to learn. Studies have shown that the infant will acknowledge the efforts of a responsive caring person rather than being commanded to react. The development of visual perception is apparent from birth, when infants are able to respond to light. During the first week the infant is naturally orientated towards the mother's face and responds preferentially to it, the infant is able to note facial expressions and is able to recognise and differentiate people at 4–6 months (Sheridan 2010).

REFLECTIVE FUNCTIONING

'Reflective functioning', described by Fonagy and Target (1997) is the uniquely human capacity to be able to make sense of one another. A parent with high reflective functioning views the infant as a separate, autonomous individual with his own thoughts and emotions and is able to understand and separate their own emotions from those of their infant. With this capacity the parent–infant relationship is strengthened and the infant learns how to understand and regulate his own behaviour. This in turn supports the infant's cognitive development. Equally the infant shares the same capacity to respond to the conception of feelings and has the ability to understand his parent's emotions. The infant projects the insecurity of their unknown emotions, such as fear or anxiety, onto their parent. The parent is able to digest these feelings and demonstrate they have the capacity to understand and interpret them, enabling them to provide a sense of calm and tranquillity. The infant is made aware of the parent's feelings towards him by reflecting and internalising the emotions his parent exhibits.

MATERNAL MENTAL HEALTH AND INFANTS

Poor maternal mental health in the perinatal period has been related to adverse outcomes for both the mother and the infant, and to parental conflict. The development of the child may be affected in several spheres, which include cognitive functioning, regulation of emotions, behavioural difficulties and psychological problems (Murray *et al.* 1996, Glover 2014, Murray 2014). Several studies have indicated the significant relation between maternal depression and impairment in bonding with the infant (McLackland *et al.* 2013, Martini *et al.* 2013). The more severe the depression, the more likely the bonding process is to be fractured (Netsi *et al.* 2014, Sockol *et al.* 2014). Depressed mothers appear to focus less on their infant, are less responsive and attuned and have difficulty synchronising their behaviour towards their infant. There is evidence that severely depressed mothers are less likely to comment appropriately on their infant's internal states, that is, what the infant might be thinking, feeling, needing or experiencing (Schacht *et al.* 2013). One possible explanation, suggested by Webb and Ayres (2014) is that mothers with depression have negative effect and cognitive biases when processing the infant's emotions.

NEUROLOGICAL STIMULATION

The importance of neurological stimulation for the infant is crucial, as recent studies have investigated the neurophysiology of the infant whose mother is depressed. There is reduced activity, particular in the frontal lobe, responsible for controlling behaviour and emotions. Changes have been found in the brain stem and mid-brain, responsible for alertness and sensation. This can result in anxiety and hyperactivity in the infant. Reduction of activity has also been found in the cortical and limbic functions, primarily responsible for emotional life and the formation of memories. This would indicate a decrease in pleasure and interest and an increase in frustration. Emotions of anger or disgust expressed by the mother therefore have a negative impact on the infant's own emotions (Martin & Markowitsch 2004). Mothers with anxiety and depression are more sensitive to negative emotions, but are also quicker to disengage from them. It is suggested that there are multiple factors which could impair bonding, which include domestic abuse, rape, poverty, making it all the more pertinent to understand the background of the parents and their socio-economic situation.

In some cultures the gender of the infant may play a part in the way in which a mother reacts to her baby and this will have an impact on maternal mental health (Patel *et al.* 2002). In Bangalore one study identified that the female infant may often act as a psycho-social stressor for the mother (Ganjekar *et al.* 2014).

SLEEP

The inability to have a satisfying sleep because of the infant's continuous crying, often caused by colic, is a challenge for both the mother and the child. Although there is little research around this area it has been found that if the infant's sleep is fragmented, there is an increased risk of the mother reporting impaired sleep, developing depressive symptoms and greater relationship stressors. In studies, the mothers' psychological well-being and sleep was greatly predicted by infants' morning saliva cortisol levels, sleep disruptions and crying intensity, whereas the duration and volume of that of the infant had a low predictive value (Kalak *et al.* 2014). The relation between maternal depressive disorders and the infant's insomnia may be explained by a transmission of unsettled maternal sleep to the foetus during pregnancy and a lack of knowledge on adequate sleep management in mothers with a previous episode of depression (St James-Roberts 2012, Martini *et al.* 2013, Petzoldt *et al.* 2014).

NEONATAL UNIT

In the USA, Segre *et al.* (2013*)* studied the benefits of listening to mothers who had a premature infant and found that during a series of personal sessions with a NICU nurse, the mothers reported lower anxiety and symptoms of depression, while their self-esteem improved. The first sessions focused on the birth of their baby and as these infants were premature, they were often taken directly to the intensive care unit and away from the mother. The mothers appreciated the fact that someone wanted to understand the emotional turmoil they experienced when separated from their poorly infant. Subsequent sessions focused on the mother herself and her needs. Often the mothers felt their well-being was secondary to that of their infant and admitted to suffering in silence as they were reluctant to discuss how they really felt. The assessments of mood and well-being which were made prior to and following the listening interventions clearly demonstrated significant improvement in the levels of both anxiety and depression, which continued to improve one month later.

However, not every depressed mother will readily report difficulty managing or connecting with her infant, thus emphasising the need to acknowledge the sentiments of impaired bonding and to possess a sound knowledge of the most effective interventions which will improve this dyadic bonding. There are many interventions which aim to increase empathic attunement and enhance secure attachment and reflective-function, some concentrating on individual therapeutic interventions and others suggesting the involvement of multi agencies to support both the mother and the infant (McLackland *et al.* 2013, Grainger & Gasson 2014). Community-based schemes appear to be more acceptable as they are more accessible and less stigmatising. The therapeutic intervention can be the remit of any assigned health worker, as some studies have suggested the occupational therapist is well placed to deliver this service (Tan & Lim 2014).

THERAPEUTIC PROGRAMMES

There are several paradigms which may be utilised to make these programmes more acceptable. These may include play, baby massage, lullabies, music, videos and the use of imaginative objects. Art as a therapy has helped mothers to develop visual language through metaphor and symbolism, expressed through the art. It was found that the process of mother–infant art therapy strengthened the emotional capacity and formation of identity of the relationship, through collaborative art production. Where the infant was encouraged to lead the dyadic dance of mark-making this enhanced the attachment and maternal sensitivity, which also helped the mother's understanding of the developmental needs of her infant and parenting capacity (Rees & Seneviratne 2014).

Many of the programmes focus on the interactions which help to enhance the development of the infant brain, promote awareness of infant cues and understand the differing cries and sounds. All are designed to not only engage the mother, but to also target the couple dyad, to ensure a secure attachment bond, and create a sound social support network that can act as a buffer for both parents against stressful situations. This awareness will ensure a sound foundation for the family to grow and develop together (Ayers *et al.* 2014, Kerstis *et al.* 2014).

Reciprocity is a strong determining factor of human behaviour and is present from birth. It is an interactive condition in which two individuals, i.e. parent and infant, mutually respond to each other while performing activities together (Fehr & Gachter 2000, Douglas & Brennan 2004). This process involves matching similar behaviours and rewarding each other with smiles, eye contact and positive reinforcement. It is essential to ensure that both the parent and infant attain the same outcomes.

Listening to infants requires being attentive to the infant's needs, by being perceptive and observing non-verbal cues and body language. The use of listening skills allows the child to hear and interpret information delivered orally and requires the child to understand the information and then respond. Sensations become perception when they are connected with stored information which allows them to take on meaning. Infants acquire language from watching, but it is a more complex process than that, as it encompasses a range of factors which include the biological make-up, cognition, psycho-social aspects and the environment in which they live.

ENVIRONMENT

As with all communicating and listening, the environment has to be appropriate. Loud music or noises from televisions can be just as disruptive for concentration for infants as it is for mothers. Therefore it is important to minimise noise. The method of delivery is important as intonation, and inflections of the voice, coupled with facial expressions, convey many meanings and as is apparent from good listening skills, infants will be able to identify if the listener is insincere. There are challenges with the depressed parent as their own communication skills may be impoverished and there might be a tendency to make negative comments, for example the parent may suggest that the infant is 'difficult to console' or 'hard to engage'. There may be a tendency for the health worker to suggest the reasons are that he is a 'demanding' or 'awkward' baby which will only serve to reinforce that the baby's expression of needs are unwarranted. Therefore extra vigilance is required to help the process with more emphasis on the achievements.

GETTING STARTED

The first introductory steps to help the parent–infant relationship are to enquire about the name of the infant, how his name was chosen, who he looks like and why. Observing and helping to guide the interactions between the two will allow the parent to be aware of behaviours they might previously have ignored. Noting the infant's response on being greeted by the parent should provide an instant impression of the relationship between the two. While the infant is making an effort to look at his mother, it is important to bring this to the mother's attention and ask why she thinks he is doing this and how she feels when she looks at him. A sense of competence can be encouraged by highlighting the fact that the infant feels safe as the parent allows them to interact within their world. This simple event can be dismissed, and the minutiae of the interaction is often unnoticed by the parent, who may rely on every nuance to make her feel capable. Directing the parent to this positive exchange can help her to realise that they are communicating. Statements like 'wow, he really likes his mum' or 'look at him smiling at you' can help to identify this.

Although the infant may be unable to vocalise, encouraging the parent to notice and to respond to whatever action he uses, for example stretching his arms and legs, by talking to him at every opportunity, saying things like 'Oh who is a tired boy?' or 'What are you doing with those arms?', can be therapeutic for both of them. However, actions may be interpreted differently, to suggest that the infant is pushing her away as he doesn't like her. Suggesting to the depressed mother that the use of actions and facial gestures when engaging with her infant helps her infant to understand what she is trying to communicate, can also be beneficial to the mother as the response she receives will affirm her abilities.

Taking time to listen to the silences and allowing the infant to assimilate the information by not rushing into the next activity or using being garrulous is also a skill. However, with the mother whose mood may be euphoric or euthymic this may present a challenge, as initially you may have to employ calming techniques to enable the parent to focus on her infant.

The ability to respond to an infant in a natural, empathetic way is often denied to the parent with depressive symptoms, who may be overwhelmed with the complexities of poor self-esteem, low expectations and other negative emotions. Some might find parenting complex, particularly when they lack support, a role model and/or have symptoms of depression and/or anxiety. It is difficult to contend with their own inabilities and sometimes this can be over-whelming, coupled with the needs and requirements of their infant. Parents may find it difficult to be sensitive to the infant's cues and the complex process of mutual regulation. As a result the depressed parent is more likely to have an impaired relationship with the infant. This interference with positive parental–infant interaction and secure attachment is disrupted, which is associated with the infant's poor social interactions and lower cognitive development when older. Some may find it demanding to relate to their infant because of traumatic events or an unexpected pregnancy, but it is only by listening to the parent that the deeper reasons for the difficulties can be exposed.

Perinatal depression and anxiety are potentially modifiable risk factors for cognitive, behavioural and emotional problems among the offspring. Studies have shown that the adverse effects on the infant seem to be long term, arguing the case that there are considerable mental health gains when the importance of parent–infant attachment is acknowledged. Therapeutic interventions focus directly on helping the parent to increase sensitivity towards her infant to help form a more positive maternal attachment (Hossein Etezady & Davis 2012). The complexity of the psychology of infants and adults continues to offer a fascinating insight into the development of human behaviour and constructs.

REFERENCES

Ayers, S., Jessup, D., Pike, A., Parfitt, Y. & Ford, E. (2014). The role of adult attachment style, birth intervention and support in posttraumatic stress after childbirth: A prospective study. *Journal of Affective Disorders* 155:295–298

Douglas, H. & Brennan, A. (2004). Containment, reciprocity and behaviour management: Preliminary evaluation of a brief earl intervention (the Solihull Approach) for families with infants and young children. *The International Journal of Infant Observation.* 7(1):89–107

Fehr, E., & Gachter, S. (2000). Fairness and retaliation: The economics of reciprocity. *Journal of Economic Perspectives* 14(3):159–181

Fonagy, P. & Target, M. (1997). *Attachment and Reflective Function: Their Role in Self-organization.* USA: Cambridge University Press

Ganjekar, S., Ramaiah, M.S., Nanjundappa, G.B., Desai, G. & Chandra, P.S. (2014). Gender of the child and psychopathology in maternal mental illness. In Abstracts for the International Marce Society for Perinatal Mental Health Biennial Scientific Conference. *Archives of Women's Mental Health* 18(2):295 published online April 2015

Glover, V. (2014). Maternal depression, anxiety and stress during pregnancy and child outcome; what needs to be done. Best Practice & Research. *Clinical Obstetrics & Gynaecology* 28:25–35

Grainger, H. & Gasson, E. (2014). Therapeutic group programme linked with nursery nurse input. In Abstracts for the International Marce Society for Perinatal Mental Health Biennial Scientific Conference. *Archives of Women's Mental Health* 18(2) published online April 2015

Hossein Etezady, M. & Davis, M. (eds) (2012).*Clinical Perspectives on Reflective Parenting: Keeping the Child's Mind in Mind.* Lanham, Maryland: Jason Aronson Inc.

Kalak, N., Brand, S., Furlano, R., Sidler, M., Schulz, J. & Holsboer-Trachsler, E. (2014). Associations between infants' crying, sleep and cortisol secretion and mother's sleep and well-being. In Abstracts for the International Marce Society for Perinatal Mental Health Biennial Scientific Conference. *Archives of Women's Mental Health* 18(2):406 published online April 2015

Kerstis, B., Berglund, A., Engstrom, G., Edlund, N., Sylven, S. & Aarts, C. (2014). Depressive symptoms postpartum among parents are associated with marital separation: A Swedish cohort study. *Scandinavian Journal of Public Health* published online 22 July 2014 DOI: 10.1177/1403494814542262: 1–9

Martin, P. & Markowitsch, H.J. (2004). Pioneers of affective neuroscience and early concepts of the emotional brain. *Journal of the History of the Neurosciences: Basic and Clinical Perspectives,* 10(1):58–66

Martini, J., Wittich, J., Petzoldt, J., Winkel, S., Einsle, F., Siegert, J., Höfler, M., Beesdo-Baum, K. & Wittchen, H-U. (2013). Maternal anxiety disorders prior to conception, psychopathology during pregnancy and early infants' development: a prospective-longitudinal study. *Archives of Womens Mental Health* 16(6):549–560

McLackland, B., Channon, S., Fowles, K. & Jones, L. (2013). An intervention aimed at helping parents with their emotional attunement to their child. *Community Practitioner* 86(4):24–27

Murray, L. (2014). *The Psychology of Babies.* London: Robinson

Murray, L., Fiori-Cowley, A., Hooper, R. & Cooper, P. (1996). The impact of postnatal depression and associated adversity on early mother-infant interactions and later infant outcome. *Child Development* 67:2512–2526

Netsi, E., Evans, J., O'Mahen, H. & Ramchandani, P. (2014). A pilot randomized controlled trial of cognitive behavioural therapy for women with antenatal depression: Infant temperament and sleep. In Abstracts for the International Marce Society for Perinatal Mental Health Biennial Scientific Conference. *Archives of Women's Mental Health* 18(2):400 published online April 2015

Patel, V., Rodrigues, M. & De Souza, N. (2002). Gender, poverty and postnatal depression: a study of mothers in Goa, India. *American Journal of Psychiatry* 159:43–47.

Petzoldt, J., Wittchen, H.U., Wittich, J. Einsle, F., Höfler, M. & Martini, J. (2014). Maternal anxiety disorders predict excessive infant crying: a prospective longitudinal study. *Archives of Disease in Childhood* 99(9):800–806

Rees, C. & Seneviratne, T. (2014). Perinatal Psychiatry and Art Psychotherapy: Interventions on a Mother and Baby Unit. In Abstracts for the International Marce Society for Perinatal Mental Health Biennial Scientific Conference. *Archives of Women's Mental Health* 18(2) published online April 2015

Schacht, R., Hammond, L., Marks, M., Wood, B. & Conroy, S. (2013). The relation between mind-mindedness in mothers with borderline personality disorder and mental state understanding in their children. *Infant and Child Development* 22(1):68–84

Segre, L.S.,Chuffo-Siewert, R., Brock, R.L. & O'Hara, M.W. (2013). Emotional distress in mothers of preterm hospitalized infants: a feasibility trial of nurse-delivered treatment. *Journal of Perinatology* 33:924–928

Sheridan, M. (2010) *From Birth to Five Years*. Updated by Sharma, A. & Cockerill, H. London: Routledge

Sockol, L., Battle, C.L., Howard., M. & Davies, T. (2014). Correlates of impaired mother-infant bonding in a partial hospital program for perinatal women. *Archives of Women's Mental Health*, March [epub ahead of print]

St James-Roberts, I. (2012). *The Origins, Prevention and Treatment of Infant Crying and Sleep Problems: An Evidence-based Guide for Healthcare Professionals and the Families they Support.* London: Routledge

Tan, J. & Lim, A. (2014) Providing occupational therapy parenting services for perinatal women: A service description and evaluation. In Abstracts for the International Marce Society for Perinatal Mental Health Biennial Scientific Conference. *Archives of Women's Mental Health* 18(2) published online April 2015

Webb, R. & Ayres, S. (2014). Processing of infant emotion by women with symptoms of psychopathology in pregnancy or after birth: A systematic review. In Abstracts for the International Marce Society for Perinatal Mental Health Biennial Scientific Conference. *Archives of Women's Mental Health* 18(2) published online April 2015

CULTURAL EXPERIENCES

7

PARENTS FROM ETHNIC MINORITY COMMUNITIES

The expansion of global economic migration has meant that increasingly, health workers have to relate to the needs of parents from ethnic minorities. Although there are a significant number of British born and educated parents within the United Kingdom (UK), some parents may actively prefer to associate with their cultural customs and choose to adopt traditional methods of child rearing. Others may embrace some of the Western conventions and decide to not to breastfeed or return to work shortly following the birth.

In the UK an estimated 5 per cent of the population originates from other countries, with the largest ethnic minority group from the Indian subcontinent, which, at 1.4 million (2.5 per cent) represents just over half the ethnic minority population. People of Afro-Caribbean and African origin make up a further quarter of the ethnic minority population, while the number of economic migrants from Europe and asylum seekers from conflicts in countries of Africa and the Middle East are increasing in numbers (ONS 2011). The knowledge and attitudes of the parents will be dependent on the length of time they have been established within the community and the influences it exerts on them. This presents the health worker with sometimes significant challenges, as the country origin of parents will differ in each area. As an example, the highest rate of teenage pregnancy in the world is reputedly in sub-Saharan Africa where girls tend to marry at an early age (Manarch *et al.* 2013).

It would be helpful to the health worker to have a sound knowledge of the current resources available within each area and the primary attitudes towards childbirth and child rearing. Migrant status has been found to be a risk factor for postpartum depressive symptomatology. Perinatal mental illness is three times more prevalent in low- and middle-income areas than in high-income areas. Yet, in the low- and middle-income settings, over approximately three-quarters of mothers are unable to access the care and treatment they need. The disabling effects on parents have been extensively researched. The negative consequences for infants' cognitive, emotional and physical health have been well documented.

Throughout most of the world pregnancy is considered a rite of passage. As a 'giver of life' the pregnant woman is regarded as the most powerful, as it is she who guarantees the future generations. She is revered, unavailable and safe, but according to myths and legends also feared because she could be ritually unclean.

It is difficult to be specific about the rites of passage, though there are generalities which are repeated across the world. In some African and Indian societies a rite of passage into adulthood is honoured by elders who initiate adolescents into the importance of moral instruction and social responsibility. The birth of an infant is regarded as a gift and in some pluralistic societies it is the responsibility of the community to determine the infant's unique qualities and trajectory through life, by using traditional rituals and birth charts.

In Poland there are, as in other European countries, superstitions around childbirth. A familiar belief is that should a mother look at an ugly person during pregnancy she will have an ugly baby; or that she should not cross her legs or sew her own clothes in order to prevent a difficult labour. Generally, the birth of a boy is favoured over girls and infants are often named after a catholic saint and have a 'nameday' rather than a birthday (Silverman 2000).

Most traditional societies acknowledge the importance of rites of passage for the mother and her infant and initiate the three phases of: preliminary (separation); liminality (from the birth to the Christening or naming ceremony); and then post-liminality (reintroduction into the community). There will be remnants of importance to the mother and her family, but each phase will differ in gravity and strength (Van Gennep 1960). These important traits attempt to guarantee the well-being of parents and their infants, physically, emotionally and spiritually.

Although the expressions of maternal and paternal mental ill health are similar throughout the world, the interpretations are often different. In the more traditional cultures mental instability is explained as the body's possession by an evil spirit, which controls or overwhelms the person's will. The treatments for this affliction are as prescriptive as Western psycho-pharmaceutical therapies and, when prescribed by a traditional healer, are believed to be as potent. The relevance of social support is important, as the adversity caused by the possession becomes the responsibility of the community and communal efforts are made to eradicate and exorcise the spirit. The spirits are not a random collection of strange effigies but have titles, ranks and positions, and their choice of why and who to possess is elaborate and complex. In the West internal factors are culpable for perinatal mental illness, whereas in the traditional cultures the blame is externalised by a spirit (Hanley & Brown 2014).

AWARENESS

The accounts of ignorance and stigma attached to mental illness are as relevant across the globe and the narratives are often reported about cruelty and mismanagement. This often generates a reluctance to discuss any idea of mental illness as some do not want the burden of mental illness or the disgrace it can bring to the family. Equally, there is an increasing reliance on primary health care, as second and third generations of migrants understand the concepts. There is an argument for amalgamating the two treatment regimes of Western and traditional medicine and this is practised very successfully in some areas (Bugdayi *et al.* 2004, Ghubash & Eapen 2009, Hanley & Brown 2014).

Recognition and awareness can help to bridge that gap. As an example, the wearing of an amulet or excess use of kohl around the eyes can be an indication of personal protection against evil spirits. Reading Holy books or adhering to Holy laws may be a forewarning of a parent's anxiety to seek solace from a spiritual source rather than the health worker. The fumes of smouldering frankincense are reputedly used to drive out evil and reinforce good, but may also be an indication of a person's fear of being surrounded by satanic forces. Any indication that the precaution has been recognised may generate a conversation around the reasons and grounds for these preventative measures.

EXERCISE 7.1

It might be helpful to examine your own skills and attitudes towards parents from ethnic minorities and to list the ways in which you might establish a rapport.

For example:

- What are your initial thoughts when you know you have to visit a family who is non-English speaking?
  Do you feel – anxious/apprehensive/angry/deflated?
- Why do you feel this way?
  Is this because of previous experiences/prejudice/stereotyping?
- Do you have a background knowledge of their origins?
- Have you researched their country of origin?
- Do you understand their child rearing processes?
- Are you aware of the different birthing practices in the country of origin?
- Are there any rituals that must be adhered to?
- In what way are the pregnancy, birth and first days regarded as a rite of passage?
- What are the expectations for breastfeeding?
- Are you aware of their support networks and who would be the most important person to help them?
- Have you visited or contacted the local place of worship/social club/specialist supermarket?
- Do you know any words in their language?

Most authorities will use professional translators to convey questions and conversations. This requires planning as the translator has to be available for the same appointment time and be able to locate the area. This is sometimes an expensive service and often there is a reluctance to use it. A translator may also be available at the end of the telephone or by Skype.

One way of establishing a conversation is to use technology and explore the possibility of using an app or with your ipad or iphone to use *Google Translate*.

An example of some of the phrases you might start with:

How are you feeling today?
You look sad.
How can I help you?
Who can you contact?
Who can I contact for you?

It is difficult to establish a rapport with parents who do not speak or find it difficult to understand English. Attempting to communicate with speech only may lead to frustration and prejudice, making assumptions about the parents' intelligence, understanding of services or ability to cope. Therefore equipped with the knowledge of patience, body language, non-verbal communication, an understanding of the cultural nuances and a few recognisable words in the parent's language, for example: 'How are you?' or 'Yes'/'No'/'Good?' 'Bad?' . . . should allow the parent to feel there is an element of empathy between the two of you.

EXERCISE 7.2

These exercises are designed to help you to try to understand what it must be like for a mother to explain her problems in a language which is unfamiliar to her

Thinking about culture and non-English speaking parents

In a group of two sit facing each other. One is **A** and one is **B**

■ **A** – Try to imagine that you need to find out how to stop your baby crying in the evenings. Do not use any words other than 'rhubarb' and 'yellow'.
■ **B** – You must try to understand what she is attempting to tell you.

This exercise should last three minutes.

EXERCISE 7.3

Thinking about culture and non-English speaking parents

During this exercise, A is unaware of B's intentions

- **A:** Does not speak English but seems upset and starts to cry.
- **B:** Try to establish what is wrong with **A**, without the use of a translator, for three minutes.
- Both feedback what this experience has meant to you.
- Did **A** feel listened to?

These exercises help to demonstrate how both the Listener and the Talker may find this exercise frustrating but also may find a sense of empathy and compassion, by the use of gestures and gesticulation which might encourage the Talker to pursue the interaction.

GLOBAL MATERNAL AND PATERNAL MENTAL HEALTH

Maternal and child health are currently key Millennium Development Goals which define the global health and development agenda (Patel 2014). There is now significant evidence to assess the relevance of maternal and paternal mental health, on not only those in high-income settings, but those parents in the low resource areas. There are global innovative practices to improve access to good mental health care and schemes highlighting the importance of integrating mental as well as physical health care into the public agenda.

A selection of the many global studies is an indicator of the current research undertaken as the popularity of perinatal mental health has a greater grasp now than it ever has. The commonality of the findings is the influence maternal mood disorder has on the health of the infant, but also that it becomes a burden on society, particularly in the developing world. It is estimated that 80 per cent of women who experience severe mental disorders live in low- and middle-income countries, where fertility rates are high and access to mental health care is limited.

In a recent systematic review of motherhood experiences of women with severe mental disorders by Boyle *et al.* (2014), all the studies identified were from high-income countries. In order to address the research gap Boyle *et al.* (2014) conducted an exploratory study in Malawi, Africa. They found that the parenting experiences of women with severe mental illness were affected by not only their mental health but others' reaction towards them within the community. Work in rural Vietnam by Tran *et al.* (2013, 2014) found that in the areas where there were high levels of financial poverty, the social and emotional development of infants was affected by the mother's mental status. The studies done by Hanlon *et al.* (2009) and Ross *et al.* (2011), however, found that maternal mental ill health in rural Ethiopia was not associated with low income and resource constrained settings, but was more likely to be associated with adverse public health outcomes for both the mother and the infant.

In South Africa van Heyningen and Honikman (2014) developed a brief mental health screening tool which was the first measure of common perinatal mental health disorders to include both mood and anxiety symptoms as well as psychological risk factors. It was intended for the use of women in low income, primary care maternity settings and was aimed at early identification of mental health risks during the perinatal period and can be used by non-specialist health care workers. Penehira and Doherty (2012) used Hoki Ki Te Rito or Mellow Parenting, which is a parenting programme using attachment theory and cognitive behavioural methods to promote change and improve parent–child interaction. The key techniques are video feedback and group dynamics which are used throughout the group-based intervention. This methodology has been found to be useful for improving the well being for Maori parents and has offered positive developmental outcomes for their infants.

In some societies gender is recognised as having a significant impact on the mental health of parents.

A study in Mexico by Asuncion *et al.* (2014) found that female gender role traditionalism increased the risk of postnatal depressive symptoms, suggesting that the expansion of the female role options, by advocating greater opportunities for women and reinforcing assertive behaviours, can be of some benefit towards preventing postnatal depression. Saeb *et al.* (2014) studied early trauma and stressful life events for the pregnant women who gave birth in a city in Mexico. The population was subjected to murders, kidnappings, shootings, armed robberies and death threats. They found the mothers were in a high risk group for depressive symptoms within the early postnatal period because of the impact of the community violence and other variables.

Mothers in Japan with anxiety and depressive symptoms demonstrated poor mother–infant interaction, and their infants showed early signs of reduced social responsiveness. It was found that they were related to both individual infant differences and a lack of maternal sensitivity to engage in social interactions. Blöchlinger *et al.* (2014), in their Swiss study, recognised the importance of a supportive midwife who provided mutual trust and was perceptive of the needs of the family. As maternal depression has a negative impact on prenatal attachment, Rubertsson *et al.* (2014) in their Swedish study recommended that there is a conversation between the midwife and the woman to understand her relationship with and attachment to her unborn child. It was suggested that this could be the first step to detecting any emotional or depressive symptoms, while being prepared to refer to longer-term counselling or support systems for both the mother and child.

In France an early pregnancy interview of both future parents by health professionals is a state recommendation (Glangeaud 2014). By offering ambulatory services which involve intensive home visiting and collaboration with other health professionals, researchers in Belgium found a significant decrease in the hospitalisation of mothers with severe mental illness (Mertens & Bauters 2014). Latina mothers in America are estimated to have three times the rate of postnatal depression of the general population. Researchers sought to refine the possible causes by identifying specific cultural and contextual frameworks which were initiated though immigration and trauma. Results from a study by Lara-Cinisomo *et al.* (2014) suggest that Latinas' treatment preferences consist of a pathway (i.e., hierarchical) approach, beginning with their personal resources, followed by more formal support systems. This included home visiting by a nurse or health professional and supplemented with behavioural therapy. Antidepressant use was judged to be acceptable only in severe cases or after delivery. In order to increase health-seeking behaviours among the Latina women it was suggested that health practitioners should first build a trusting relationship.

It has been speculated that women of South Asian origin have a higher prevalence of depression in comparison with their white counterparts. Several studies have been carried out in the United Kingdom and the West, to ascertain the attitudes towards postnatal depression of women from Bangladesh and Pakistan (Downe *et al.* 2007, Baldwin & Griffiths 2009, Nilaweera *et al.* 2014). Some studies have found that the language and cultural awareness form some of the barriers which make access to this community difficult. Lack of education has meant that some health workers are reluctant to engage with parents, particularly with issues concerning mental illness. Even in the West, mothers find it difficult to access perinatal mental health services as Dennis and Chung-Lee (2006) found in their study of Canadian mothers.

A study by Husain *et al.* (2012) demonstrated that using culturally sensitive and adapted interventions which were underpinned by using cognitive behavioural therapy, provided an acceptable resource for the British South Asian mothers suffering from postpartum mental disorders. Hasan (2014) reported that following the readings of the *Holy Quran* and the *Sunnah* suggests that the act of breastfeeding elevates the status of the mother and it is advised to breastfeed for two years to create an attachment between the mother and baby which aids the improvement of physical, psychological development and socialisation skills (Yusuf 2014). Husain *et al.* (2012) found other main concerns which included trust issues and stigma. It was also noted that there was a lack of access to support services. In a Canadian study Zelkowitz *et al.* (2008) found there was less psychological stress with the immigrant population than with those born in Canada, which suggested a 'health migrant' effect and was perhaps related to cultural norms.

Screening and assessment is recommended by the International Marcé Society for Perinatal Mental Health (Austin & Hanley 2013). It is also recommended in Italy and Banti *et al.* (2011) in their study recognised that it can reduce the rates of perinatal psychopathology and detect women at the highest risk of developing perinatal depression, allowing an earlier diagnosis and a better treatment management. In Turkey follow-up studies by Akcali Aslan *et al.* (2014) and Kirkan *et al.* (2014) established that untreated depression is an important predictor for postpartum depression. They advocated the importance of screening in the antenatal period and the need for access for psychiatric treatment as necessary.

The Nordic countries present unique opportunities to perform population-based studies because of their public health care systems. They are ideally suited for studies on child and parental mental health (Garthus-Niegel *et al.* 2013). The Nordic health care system has a well-established heritage in primary and preventive health care. Local child health care centres have been established for over 70 years and provide routine health-control examinations free of charge for all children from birth through six years of age. In a study in Finland by Mäki *et al.* (2010) it was found that mothers who had antenatal depression had a slightly increased risk of depression in their children when compared with mothers who did not suffer from depression. It was found that antenatal depression may act as an adverse environmental factor for those with a genetic vulnerability.

Turkey has the highest pregnancy rate in Europe. A Turkish prospective population-based study by Yuce *et al.* (2014) and Kirkan *et al.* (2014) evaluated the frequency of denial of pregnancy. The denial of pregnancy throughout most of gestation has significant risks to both mother and foetus because of inadequate prenatal care, poor nutrition, foetal abuse, unattended or precipitous delivery. It was found that the occurrence of denied pregnancy appeared to be similar across different socio-demographic conditions, negating the view that denial of pregnancy is a rare event. Psychiatrists face the dilemma of treating depressed pregnant women with medication because of the impact on the foetus and early childhood growth. The study compared women with major depression who were treated with antidepressants, untreated women with major depression and healthy women during pregnancy with respect to birth weight and preterm birth in Turkey. The results suggested that mothers with major depression during pregnancy had newborns with lower birth weights and shorter lengths of gestation compared with non-depressed ones. Antidepressant treatment of major depression during pregnancy is unrelated to increased risk of shorter gestational age and lower birth weight. Therefore awareness is necessary for prevention of unwanted consequences.

This plethora of emerging global research is encouraging, highlighting not only the similarities in symptomatic features, risk factors and consequences of perinatal mental health, but also amalgamating the differing treatment and management options for parents and their infants. Whatever the race, class or creed the impact of perinatal mental health remains constant. Therefore maintaining the good mental health of women and fathers should be a major consideration worldwide.

REFERENCES

Akcali Aslan P., Aydin, N. Yazici, E., Aksoy, A.N., Kirkan, T.S. & Daloglu, G.A. (2014). Prevalence of depressive disorders and related factors in women in the first trimester of their pregnancies in Erzurum, Turkey. *International Journal of Social Psychiatry.* Feb 26

Asuncion, L., Navarrete, L. & Nieto, L. (2014). The Impact of Female Gender Role Traditionalism in Postpartum Depression. In Abstracts for the International Marce Society for Perinatal Mental Health Biennial Scientific Conference. *Archives of Women's Mental Health* 18(2):304 published online April 2015

Austin, M.P. & Hanley, J. (2013). Perinatal psychosocial assessment and depression screening. *Journal of Health Visiting* 1(10):550

Baldwin, S. & Griffiths, P. (2009). Do specialist community public health nurses assess risk factors for depression, suicide, and self-harm among south Asian mothers living in London? *Public Health Nurse* 26(3):277–289

Banti, S., Mauri, M. Oppo, A., Borri, C., Rambelli, C., Ramacciotti, D., Montagnani, M.S., Camilleri, V., Cortopassi, S., Rucci, P. & Cassano, G.B. (2011). From the third month of pregnancy to 1 year postpartum. Prevalence, incidence, recurrence, and new onset of depression. Results from the Perinatal Depression–Research & Screening Unit study. *Comprehensive Psychiatry* 52:343–351

Blöchlinger, P., Kurth, E. & Frei, I.A. (2014) What women want: a qualitative study about postnatal midwifery care at home. In Abstracts for the International Marce Society for Perinatal Mental Health Biennial Scientific Conference. *Archives of Women's Mental Health* 18(2):321 published online April 2015

Boyle, E., Stewart, R.C. & Davis, J. (2014). An exploratory study of the childbearing and parenting experiences of women with severe mental disorders in Malawi. In Abstracts for the International Marce Society for Perinatal Mental Health Biennial Scientific Conference. *Archives of Women's Mental Health* 18(2):358 published online April 2015

Bugdayi, R., Sanmaiz, C.T., Tezcanm, H., Kurt, A.O. & Oner, S. (2004). A cross sectional prevalence study of depression at various times after delivery in Mesin Province in Turkey. *Journal of Women's Health* 13(1):63–68 Jan–Feb

Dennis, C-L. & Chung-Lee, L. (2006). Postpartum depression help-seeking behaviours and treatment preferences: A qualitative systematic review. *Birth* 33:323–331

Downe, S., Butler, E. & Hinder, S. (2007). Screening tools for depressed mood after childbirth in UK-based south Asian women: A systematic review. *Journal of Advanced Nursing* 57(6):565–583

Garthus-Niegel, S., von Soest, T., Vollrath, M.E. & Eberhard-Gran, M. (2013). The impact of subjective birth experiences on post-traumatic stress symptoms: a longitudinal study. *Archives of Women's Mental Health* 16:1–10

Ghubash, R. & Eapen, V. (2009) Postpartum mental illness; perspectives from an Arabian Gulf Population. *Psychological Reports* 105(1):127–136

Glangeaud, N. (2014). Mother-Baby Perinatal Treatment Impact and Management of Care in Different Countries. In Abstracts for the International Marce Society for Perinatal Mental Health Biennial Scientific Conference. *Archives of Women's Mental Health* 18(2) published online April 2015

Hanley, J. & Brown, A. (2014). Cultural variations in interpretation of postnatal illness: Jinn possession among Muslim communities. *Community Mental Health Journal* Apr 50(3):348–353. doi: 10.1007/s10597–013–9640–4. Epub 2013 Aug 17

Hanlon, C., Medhin, G., Alem, A., Tesfaye, F., Lakew, Z., Worku, B., Dewey, M., Araya, M., Abdulahi, A., Hughes, M., Tomlinson, M., Patel, V. & Prince, M. (2009). Impact of antenatal common mental disorders upon perinatal outcomes in Ethiopia: the P-MaMiE population-based cohort study. *Tropical Medicine and International Health* 14:156–166

Hasan, N. (2014). The Quranic recommendation on breast feeding. In Abstracts for the International Marce Society for Perinatal Mental Health Biennial Scientific Conference. *Archives of Women's Mental Health* 18(2) published online April 2015

Husain, N., Cruickshank, K., Husain, M., Khan, S., Tomenson, B. & Rahman, A. (2012). Social stress and depression during pregnancy and in the postnatal period in British Pakistani mothers: a cohort study. *Journal of Affective Disorders* Nov 140(3):268–276

Kirkan, T.S., Aydin, N., Yazici, E., Akcali Aslan, P., Acemoglu, H. & Daloglu, A.G. (2014). The depression in women in pregnancy and postpartum period: A follow-up study. *International Journal of Social Psychiatry* Jul 27

Lara-Cinisomo, S. *et al.* (2014). Perinatal depression treatment preferences among Latina mothers. *Qualitative Health Research* 24(2):232–241

Mäki, P., Riekki, T., Miettunen, J., Isohanni, M., Jones, P.B., Murray, G.K. & Veijola, J. (2010). Schizophrenia in the offspring of antenatally depressed mothers in the Northern Finland 1966 Birth Cohort – relationship to family history of psychosis. *American Journal of Psychiatry* 167:70–77

Manarch, M., Long, M. & Casey, P. (2013). Current issues in contraception. *May Clinic Proceedings* 88(3):295–299

Mertens, C. & Bauters, K. (2014). Integrated and modular treatment of postpartum problems in Ghent (Flandres – Belgium). In Abstracts for the International Marce Society for Perinatal Mental Health Biennial Scientific Conference. *Archives of Women's Mental Health* 18(2):364 published online April 2015

Nilaweera, I., Doran, F. & Fisher, J. (2014). Prevalence, nature and determinants of postpartum mental health problems among women who have migrated from south Asian to high-income countries: A systematic review of the evidence. *Journal of Affective Disorders* 166:213–226

Office of National Statistics. (2011). KS201UK Ethnic group, local authorities in the United Kingdom

Patel, V. (2014). Maternal mental health and global health. The Channi Kumar lecture. In Abstracts for the International Marce Society for Perinatal Mental Health Biennial Scientific Conference. *Archives of Women's Mental Health* 18(2) published online April 2015

Penehira, M. & Doherty, L. (2012). Tu mai te oriori, nau mai te hauora! A kaupapa Māori approach to infant mental health: Adapting Mellow Parenting for Māori mothers in Aotearoa, New Zealand. Pimatisiwin *A Journal of Aboriginal & Indigenous Community Health* 10(3):367–382

Ross, J., Hanlon, C., Medhin, G., Alem, A., Tesfaye, F., Worku, B., Dewey, M., Patel, V. & Prince, M. (2011). Perinatal mental distress and infant morbidity in Ethiopia: a cohort study. *Archives of Disease in Childhood. Fetal and Neonatal Edition* 96:F59–64

Rubertsson, C., Haines, H., Sydsjö, G., Pallant, J., Hildingsson, I, & Cross, M. (2014). Psychometric evaluation and refinement of the Prenatal Attachment Inventory. *Journal of Reproductive and Infant Psychology* DOI:10.1080/02646838.2013.871627

Saeb, S., Subirà, S., Gelabert, E., Torres, A., Martin-Santos, R. & Garcia-Esteve, L. (2014). Traumatic experiences and postpartum depressive symptoms in

Mexican women. In Abstracts for the International Marce Society for Perinatal Mental Health Biennial Scientific Conference. *Archives of Women's Mental Health* 18(2):343 published online April 2015

Silverman, D. (2000). *Polish American Folklore.* Urbana & Chicago: University of Illinois Press

Tran, T., Biggs, B.A., Simpson, J., Tran, T.D., Hanieh, S., Dwyer, T. & Fisher, J. (2013). Impact on infants' cognitive development of antenatal exposure to iron deficiency disorder and common mental disorders. *PLOS One* 8(9):1–9 e74876

Tran, T.D., Biggs, B.A, Tran, T., Simpson, J.A, Cabral de Mello, M., Hanieh, S., Nguyen, T.T., Dwyer, T.& Fisher J. (2014). Perinatal common mental disorders among women and the social and emotional development of their infants in rural Vietnam. *Journal of Affective Disorders* 160:104–112

Van Gennep (1960). *The Rites of Passage.* London: Routledge (reprinted 2004)

Van Heyningen & Honikman, S. (2014). Development of a mental health screening instrument for use in low-resource, primary care, antenatal settings in South Africa. In Abstracts for the International Marce Society for Perinatal Mental Health Biennial Scientific Conference. *Archives of Women's Mental Health* 18(2):304 published online April 2015

Yuce, H., Aydin, N., Omay, O., Kosan, Z., Gultekin, A.G., Aksoy, A. & Wessel, J. (2014). Prevalence of denial of pregnancy and associated factors in Turkey. In Abstracts for the International Marce Society for Perinatal Mental Health Biennial Scientific Conference. *Archives of Women's Mental Health* 18(2):394 published online April 2015

Yusuf, A.A. *The Holy Quran translation and commentary,* Chapters 2:233; 31:14; 28:7, 12, 13; 46:15; 65:6; 4:23. Middlesex, HA2 8JQ UK: Islamic Propagation Centre International

Zelkowitz, P., Saucier, J.F., Wang, T., Katofsky, L., Valenzuela, M. & Westreich, R. (2008). Stability and change in depressive symptoms from pregnancy to two months postpartum in childbearing immigrant women. *Archives of Women's Mental Health* 11:1–11

8

RESOURCES AND LOOKING AFTER YOURSELF

'It is the disease of not listening, the malady of not marking that I am troubled withal'

(Henry IV Part 1 act 5 sc 1, 1. Shakespeare)

Listening is a powerful, compassionate skill but it is also complex and demanding and can quickly deplete your energy levels. It would not be unusual to complete a visit feeling exhausted. You will have spent an hour being attentive to someone else's need. Devoid of your own self-interest, you will shift between tranquillity and composure to stress and anxiety, as you try to make sense of and understand someone else's pain and misery without absorbing all the emotional turmoil. Hearing, understanding and then feeding back are the key elements to the skill of listening. Feeding back the thoughts and feelings in small sensitive chunks allows you to leave the parent with a solution focus and therefore sense of ownership of the problem. This should free you up to become more creative and enthusiastic to deal with the next challenge.

There are times when you may feel deflated, depleted, with episodes of self-doubt, wondering what you have achieved or what, if any, progress you have made. This time allows you to process your thoughts to enable you to focus on your own development and learning needs. Seeking help or supervision can help to restore your confidence or change your approach, so that your level of stress is reduced.

SUPERVISION

There are many models of supervision or support which focus on disentangling the emotional morass which some health workers may experience. Supervision is a formative process which allows the health worker to self-assess their working practice, self-analyse the reasons for their thoughts and feelings and reflect deeply on the profundities of what may have been heard or interpreted (DoH 1993). In the case of the listening visit, it is designed to enhance the health worker's skills which in turn will benefit the parent. It can facilitate both confidence and competence in the listening process when any doubts can be expressed and rationalised. This in turn can expand the tacit knowledge base, also known as implicit knowledge, which is difficult to transfer and which you cannot accumulate by reading the literature but only by experiencing the experience of listening.

Often one type of support is insufficient and relies on the foundation of other trusted brands of psychological interventions. Restorative Clinical Supervision is a model which focuses on the capacity of the health worker to work as a supervisor, to engage in their clinical work rather than on the clinical work itself (Wallbank 2012). The model purports to build autonomy, undertake caseloads more effectively and create stronger working relationships, which inevitably reduced absenteeism in the workplace.

Kadushin (1992), in reference to Dawson (1926), outlines the three stages of supervision which are educative (formative), administrative and supportive. The educative stage focuses on instrumental needs, whereas the supportive stage is more concerned with expressed needs. The *educative* or formative development of each individual worker is through learning from the wisdom of the more experienced supervisor who can assist in analysing the observations, exploring and reflecting on the encounter in order to better understand the parent. It can help to understand the dynamics of the relationship with the parent and to explore each other's reaction and responses. Additionally the supervision can examine what interventions were used and what were the consequences of the intervention and finally it can explore different ways in which to work with the parents (Hawkins & Shohet 1989, 2007).

The *supportive* stage is less formal and relies on the attributes of the supervisor who has the ability to communicate with confidence and instil confidence in the health worker by being both available and approachable. The supervisor supports the health worker to know that although they may be working autonomously, there is a supportive network. The health worker invariably respects their opinions and is able to enhance their independent functioning, particularly if their decisions are validated and sanctioned. Supervisors are able to reduce the personal stress of the health worker by offering an objective perspective, preventing stressful situations by excusing failure, when appropriate, and help the health worker to adjust to the stress.

The *administrative* stage ensures the quality of the work remains consistent and outlines room for improvement. This stage guarantees that there is both the environment and the space to enable the health worker to express their personal distress. It is concerned more with the managerial aspects to affirm that both personal and professional resources are appropriate and available.

The normative role is similar to the administrative role, whereby during the supervision, the supervisor is expected to accept the responsibility for the health worker to ensure they adhere to and meet the organisational, ethical and professional standards and operate within the prescribed codes and laws.

Accessing supervision in the workplace can be difficult and there may be resistance to allowing absence from work in order to complete sessions, thus making it important to find ways in which to de-stress. This may be achieved in a number of ways and it is important to have someone in whom you can confide. That might be someone of a religious persuasion or a trusted friend, who will take the time to just listen to you. If you are working as a part of a team, then there will be similar requirements to have a meeting about particular cases or make provision for each member to have access to group supervision, where the object is not to compete with each other but to use the same compassion and passion as you would if listening to a parent.

LIMITATIONS

Knowing your limitations is important, as is being sufficiently perceptive to say 'No'. There is little merit in accepting more work if you are fighting to survive, but often we are unable to recognise when we are overwhelmed until it is too late. It is a skill to draw boundaries and should be regarded as an act of self-protection (Berhard 2011). There can be no value in exhausting yourself, as it is possible this will dent your confidence and it is unlikely you will be able to support others. Refusing to do something or to continue with something you feel is beyond your expertise is not a negative solution, but will protect you and often earn you respect. Offering the parent an alternative avenue of help is more likely to be of more support to them than you both labouring on trying to find a solution to the insolvable.

Good mental well-being means feeling happy about your life and having the ability to enjoy it the way you want to. Studies have shown that what we do and how we think have the biggest impact on our general well-being. It is important to connect with our bodies and the sensations we experience like the sights, sounds, tastes and smells that surround us now. As an example, sitting by the computer and being aware that you can hear the continuous hum of the machine, feel the wood of the chair against your back, smell the fresh air coming in from the open window and see the icons on the bright screen.

HELPFUL TECHNIQUES

Learning the techniques of mindfulness can help you become more aware of the present moment and discover how to enjoy it (NHS Choices 2014). Mark Williams, Professor of clinical psychology at the Oxford Mindfulness Centre is a great proponent of mindfulness and explains that it means knowing directly what is going on inside and outside ourselves, moment by moment. It is also known as *present-centredness*, and can help us enjoy the world more and understand ourselves better.

Yoga offers an excellent way of preserving your well-being. The series of movements is designed to increase your strength and flexibility. Persistence, with practice, can provide an overall feeling of well-being.

Ten years ago there would have been a dearth of services for mothers and their infants but today the growing interest in perinatal mental health has meant an explosion in the number of agencies who are taking an active interest in the condition and are passionate about making a difference. A knowledge of the available local and national services for further support is valuable. In the United Kingdom, there are several charitable and voluntary organisations emerging who will work with parents. Specialist perinatal mental health teams are continually being developed, offering consultations for mothers, fathers and infants. There are societies who encourage research into the causes of perinatal mental illness and solutions to the problems. There are internet resources which include new and exciting ways of reaching younger parents, to include apps and videos on YouTube.

Today work in the field of perinatal mental health is stimulating and motivating, but very little will move forward if we do not ask the question 'How do you feel?' and take the time to listen for the answer.

EXERCISE 8.1

Looking after yourself

- When was the last time you spoke to someone in your family about how you really feel?
- When was the last time you spoke with your friends about how you really feel?
- How long ago is it since you really treated yourself?
- What do you consider a treat? Write down the list of things that occur to you – note how many of them include time, alcohol and ablutions (having the time to drink a glass of wine while having a bath!).

Writing your thoughts down will help you to consolidate how often you seek help and what pleasures you allow yourself.

REFERENCES

Berhard, T. (2011). *Turning Straw into Gold*. Life through a Buddhist lens. www.psychologytoday.com

Dawson, J.B. (1926). The casework supervisor in a family agency. *Family* 6: 293–295

Department of Health (1993). *A vision for the future*. Report of the Chief Nursing Officer

Hawkins, P. & Shohet, R. (1989, 2007). *Supervision in the Helping Professions. An individual, group and organizational approach*. Milton Keynes: Open University Press/Maidenhead: Open University Press

Kadushin, A. (1992). *Supervision in Social Work* (3rd edn). New York: Columbia University Press. Revised fourth edition published 2002

NHS Choices. www.nhs.uk/conditions

Wallbank, S. (2012). Health visitor needs: National perspectives from the Restorative Clinical Supervision Programme. *Community Practitioner* 85(4):29–32

SCENARIOS

These scenarios are designed to be used in group work, to help make sense of what has been written. The answers are what might be seen, heard or said during the interactions.

SCENARIO ONE

Clair is an executive in a busy City bank, which is a two-hour train journey from her home. She has recently returned to work following her three months of maternity leave. Clair had an au pair to care for her baby, Oliver, but the au pair has recently given Clair very short notice to quit. Clair has had to take time off from work until she has secured another au pair. Her parents live in the country and her mother cares for her father who is suffering from dementia. Clair's husband had an affair with his secretary and left Clair a week ago.

Clair is at home when you call in the afternoon. Although she was expecting you, the house is untidy. Clair is welcoming, is in her dressing gown and smells strongly of alcohol. She seems unsteady on her feet and when she sits down starts to sob. You can hear the baby crying in the background.

- What are your first impressions?
- What are the possible positive aspects of each impression?
- What are the possible negative aspects of each impression?
- What will you do next?
- How will you proceed?

- **What are your first impressions?**

  I cannot see the baby.

- **What are the possible positive aspects?**

  You can hear Oliver crying so he must be alright.

- **What are the possible negative aspects?**

  Clair does not seem concerned with the crying.

  Oliver sounds in distress.

  The room appears to be untidy.

- **What are the possible positive aspects?**

  Clair is too preoccupied being a mother to have time to do the housework.

  Clair is unwell and cannot clean the house.

■ **What are the possible negative aspects?**

Clair does not have the energy to clean the house.

Clair does not have the interest to clean the house.

Clair cannot cope with the amount of housework she has to do.

<u>Clair is in her dressing gown.</u>

■ **What are the possible positive aspects?**

Clair might be feeling unwell and has just got out of bed.

Clair might be more comfortable in her dressing gown.

■ **What are the possible negative aspects?**

Clair does not have the energy to get dressed – she is an executive so is probably used to being smartly dressed.

<u>Clair smells strongly of drink.</u>

■ **What are the possible positive aspects?**

Clair has been taking alcohol for medicinal purposes.

■ **What are the possible negative aspects?**

It is too early in the day to start drinking.

Perhaps Clair has been drinking all day?

Clair has a problem with the amount of alcohol she drinks.

Clair is alcohol dependent.

<u>Clair is unsteady on her feet.</u>

■ **What are the possible positive aspects?**

Clair has vertigo, an ear infection or explained medical illness.

■ **What are the possible negative aspects?**

Clair has had too much to drink.

<u>Clair has started to sob.</u>

■ **What are the possible positive aspects?**

Clair is unwell and feels under the weather.

Clair has pain.

■ **What are the possible negative aspects?**

Clair is unhappy.

Claire is unable to cope.

Clair is depressed.

■ **What will you do next?**

Ask Clair if she is okay.

■ **What are the possible positive aspects?**

Clair might be appreciative of my concern.

Clair might say she is fine but is just having a bad day.

■ **What are the possible negative aspects?**

Clair might be embarrassed.

Clair might say she is fine and she was just being silly.

Ask Clair if I may sit down and talk.

■ **What are the possible positive aspects?**

Clair might appreciate the fact that I have acknowledged that I have the time for her.

■ **What are the possible negative aspects?**

Clair might feel I am being intrusive.

Claire might get angry and tell me to go.

Sit in the chair opposite Clair.

■ **What are the possible positive aspects?**

I have checked that this is the appropriate position and that I am able to touch Clair and hand her a handkerchief or tissue.

I have assumed the same level as Clair.

■ **What are the possible negative aspects?**

Clair might ask me to move as I am too close.

Clair might insist I remain standing.

Pass a handkerchief to Clair and acknowledge that she will take time to compose herself.

■ **What are the possible positive aspects?**

You are giving Clair the permission to compose herself.

You have indicated that you are not uncomfortable with her emotions.

You have indicated you have time for Clair.

■ **What are the possible negative aspects?**

You could feel uncomfortable with Clair crying and ask her to stop – saying something like – 'come on now, there is no need to cry'.

You might be unsure of how long to let her cry.

You might feel the need to make it better.

Ask Clair how she is feeling.

■ **What are the possible positive aspects?**

You have indicated that you are concerned about her and how she is feeling.

You have asked an open question and allowed her to answer what she feels.

■ **What are the possible negative aspects?**

Clair could tell you she feels fine and there is nothing for you to worry about.

Ask about Oliver and that you would like to see him.

■ **What are the possible positive aspects?**

You have asked about the baby and this indicates the importance of both his and her health.

You have allowed Clair to talk about her baby.

■ **What are the possible negative aspects?**

Clair says he is asleep and she does not want to disturb him.

■ **What will I do next?**

Once you have established a rapport with Clair, using your body language, positioning and non-verbal cues, you can with open questions determine the reason why both she and Oliver are crying.

Thinking about the minutiae of this simple visit, it can uncover a multitude of possible scenarios and recognises the skills necessary in the Listener.

The first is observation, which includes:

■ the condition of the house
■ the condition of Clair
■ the condition of Oliver

A. It is possible that Clair is coping well and that having flu, she took a drink of whiskey and lemon to soothe her cough. She sobbed because she stubbed her toe on the chair as she opened the door.

B. It is possible however that Clair was overwhelmed with:

- the demands of childcare
- lack of experience in childcare
- lack of support from her parents
- the challenge of knowing her mother needs to care for her father
- the challenge of housework
- loneliness, as she works in the City and may not know anyone locally
- lack of support from the partner
- financial restrictions

The only way to determine Clair's situation is to ask her, as it is easy to make assumptions and the easiest way is to conclude that **A** is the reason for her demeanour.

The skill is the understanding that Clair is overwhelmed by her circumstances and eliciting the reasons for this. You will now have a clear understanding of the signs and symptoms of postnatal depression and the risk factors. You will know the telltale signs of someone not coping and you will be able to understand why Clair might be angry or embarrassed by your questions.

When Clair resists your help – how can you overcome the barriers she is erecting to make you 'go away'?

To unpick some of them:

Depressive symptoms

Clair might say she is fine and she was just being silly.

You might ask Clair what she means by *being silly* – could she tell you more about this. Does she just feel silly today or is this something she has felt for a while? Has this persisted for more than a few weeks? This will help you to establish how Clair is really feeling and the extent of her sadness.

Crying

What do you feel about other people crying?

- It is okay?
- Do you allow them to cry, or try to stop them?
- When is it appropriate?
- How long should you let someone cry without interrupting?
- Should you cry with them?

These are the questions to ask yourself.

Often it is difficult to determine the length of time, but there will be a natural 'break' when you are able to intervene and ask if she is okay. There is an element of sensitivity in handing over the handkerchief as you do not want the mother to feel rushed and that she should 'dry her eyes and stop crying, as it is not good for you'.

Self-medication with alcohol

You might think about your attitude towards drinking alcohol and the reasons for doing so.

- Do you have the appropriate skills to be able to help someone with a problem with alcohol dependency?
- Do you understand the effect this has on infants?
- Do you understand the effect this has on family members?
- Do you know where and how to refer someone who requires help?

Would you feel comfortable asking the following?

- The reasons why someone has the need to drink?
- Is it to self-medicate?
- Do you drink out of habit?

How will you proceed?

You have established that Clair has depressive symptoms, is self-medicating and is finding caring for Oliver difficult.
 You can:

- suggest that Clair contact the general practitioner, to inform him of her mental health;
- discuss the care of Clair with the general practitioner;
- discuss with Clair with the possibility of four to six listening visits – here you may have the problem of Clair returning to work, so you might consider a Skype call at a convenient time where confidentiality can be assured.

Practical suggestions:

- demonstrate how Clair can engage with Oliver by responding to his verbal and non-verbal cues;
- contact numbers for childcare organisations;
- contact numbers for local maternal self-help groups;
- contact number for local Alcohol Anonymous group or other organisations which can offer help with alcohol dependence.

Suggested further information and reading

- Think about, and research, the charitable and voluntary organisations which may be able to assist in the care of Clair and Oliver.

- Explore the websites which offer self-help for Clair.
- Gain an understanding of the effect of self-medication, particularly on depressive symptoms.
- Understand the impact of alcohol consumption on the foetus and infants.
- Understand the impact of alcohol consumption on the family.
- Understand the process of depressive symptoms.

Do not assume that every health professional would ask the appropriate questions, as you will have noticed that this exercise is time consuming and often it is easier to ask fewer rather than more, investigative questions. You are aware that the time invested in both Clair and Oliver will have a significant impact on the well-being of Clair and the mental and physical development of Oliver.

SCENARIO TWO

Violet is a mixed race, slim, 16-year-old with 3-month-old twin girls, called Sunshine and Sky. She is living with a man twenty years older than her in social housing on a large inner city estate. She was fostered throughout her childhood and has little contact with her mother, a known drug addict, or her father, whom she believes lives in the West Indies, where his family reside. She worked in a local store but was made redundant when she found she was five months pregnant. The house is fully decorated and clean.

Violet has been through the EPDS with the health professional and scored highly on the questions, particularly those about her anxiety state. She has admitted that she has always been a wild child without boundaries, which is why her mother put her into care.

She has been prone to panic attacks but recently has found little joy with her infant girls and has ticked 'yes' to question 10 which referred to the fact that the thought of harming herself has occurred to her.

On further exploration of the question it was found that she was already self-harming, which was evidenced by the marks on her legs, some of which were bleeding. Violet bites her lip while she fidgets with Sunshine's dress and does not seem to listen to you.

- What are your first impressions?
- What are the possible positive aspects of each impression?
- What are the possible negative aspects of each impression?
- What will you do next?
- How will you proceed?

- **What are your first impressions?**

  The house is beautifully clean.

- **What are the possible positive aspects?**

  Violet is able to manage two babies and maintain a beautiful house, in spite of her age.

■ **What are the possible negative aspects?**

Has too much time been spent on the housework at the expense of the twins' care?

<u>Violet looks thin and pale.</u>

■ **What are the possible positive aspects?**

Violet takes care of her diet and has regained her weight prior to birth.

■ **What are the possible negative aspects?**

Violet takes insufficient time to care for herself.

Perhaps she is not eating well?

<u>Violet is very young and must have conceived the twins when she was under 16 years.</u>

■ **What are the possible positive aspects?**

It might not have been in the UK, where it would be an offence.

■ **What are the possible negative aspects?**

It is an offence in some countries to have sex with a person less than 16 years of age.

<u>The twins are immaculately dressed.</u>

■ **What are the possible positive aspects?**

The twins are very well cared for.

Violet must spend significant time washing their clothes.

■ **What are the possible negative aspects?**

Is she taking care of the twins over her own care?

Violet might be obsessed with cleanliness.

From the marks on her legs, it possibly reflects the level of her anxiety state.

■ **What will you do next?**

You have already entered into dialogue and have established that Violet requires, and has accepted, listening visits and have arranged a time for another visit.

<u>Ask Violet when she started self-harming and if she can remember why she did this.</u>

■ **What are the possible positive aspects?**

You have indicated that you are concerned about her and have an understanding of the process of self-harm.

You have asked open questions and allowed Violet to discuss the reasons for her self-harm and to reflect on the reasons why she persists in doing this.

This may open other avenues of concern – low self-esteem/abuse/domestic violence.

■ **What are the possible negative aspects?**

Violet might not know the reasons but could tell you she feels fine as she has been doing it for ages and there is nothing for you to worry about.

You might ask Violet what impact she thinks this is having on herself.

■ **What are the possible positive aspects?**

You have indicated that you are concerned about Violet's health and allowed her to talk about herself.

Violet might indicate that although she has been self-harming for several years, she has not discounted the thought of suicide.

■ **What are the possible negative aspects?**

Violet might feel that although she knows it makes a mess there is nothing she can do about it, and it is her way of coping, and nothing to do with you.

You might ask Violet what impact she thinks this is having on the twins.

■ **What are the possible positive aspects?**

Violet might not have considered that her mood state would have an effect on her twins and this will provide her with the opportunity to reflect on this.

■ **What are the possible negative aspects?**

Violet might be concerned that you are threatening the care of her twins and that you are looking for excuses to take her children into care.

You might ask Violet what support she has.

■ **What are the possible positive aspects?**

You are allowing Violet to consider her support network and her relationship with her parents.

Violet might confess that:

–   she feels isolated, with a poor support network, which consists mostly of her partner's older friends;

–   she feels lonely as she misses her father and wishes she had a firmer relationship with her mother.

■ What are the possible negative aspects?

Violet might feel you are examining her coping abilities and once again feel that you are exploring the possibilities of taking her children into care.

Even though a rapport has been established with Violet, using your body language, positioning and non-verbal cues and open questions, Violet may still be threatened by your presence and feel you are there to judge her. It is important that you remember person-centred, non-judgemental listening and do not make hasty decisions based on a risk assessment of safeguarding issues.

If you allow Violet to tell her story and listen to what she has to say, you may find it is a different scenario from the child protection route. Remember some mothers with mental health problems have complained that statutory services were too quick to take the children into care without understanding the whole situation. This does not mean you reject any thought of safeguarding the twins, but give due consideration to the needs of both Violet and the twins.

The first is observation, which includes:

■   the condition of the house
■   the condition of Violet
■   the condition of the twins

It is possible however that Violet has:

■   suffered from low self-esteem
■   safeguarding issues
■   traits of obsessive compulsive disorder (OCD)
■   a history of self-harm
■   been subjected to domestic abuse
■   a lack of experience in childcare
■   a lack of any support from her parents
■   the challenge of housework
■   loneliness

The only way to determine Violet's circumstances is to ask her, as it is easy to make assumptions and to conclude that this is a safeguarding issue alone.

The skill is the understanding that Violet might be overwhelmed by her circumstances and eliciting the reasons for this. You will now have a clear understanding of the signs and symptoms of obsessive compulsive disorder and the associated risk factors. You will know the telltale signs of someone not coping and you will be able to understand why Violet might be threatened by your questions.

When Violet feels threatened by you – how can you assure her that you are there to help and listen and not to judge?

How will you proceed?

You have established that Violet has OCD, is self-harming, is anxious and has poor self-esteem and might have been subjected to abuse. Although she cares for her twins she is more concerned with their outward appearance and less concerned with their developmental and mental well-being.

You can:

- suggest that Violet contact the general practitioner, to inform him of her mental health;
- discuss the care of Violet with the general practitioner;
- discuss the care of Violet with social services;
- suggest that you visit Violet for listening visits;
- examine your thoughts about safeguarding;
- examine your thoughts about self-harm.

Practical suggestions:

- demonstrate how Violet can engage with the twins by responding to their verbal and non-verbal cues;
- contact numbers and websites for OCD groups;
- contact numbers for local maternal self-help groups.

Suggested further information and reading

- Think about, and research, the charitable and voluntary organisations which may be able to assist in the care of Violet and the twins.
- Explore the websites which offer self-help for Violet.
- Gain an understanding of OCD and anxiety and the process of this.
- Understand the impact of anxiety and OCD on the foetus and infants.
- Understand the impact of anxiety and OCD on the family.
- Understand the process of safeguarding children in your area.

Do not assume that every health professional would ask the appropriate questions as you will have noticed that this exercise is time-consuming and often it is easier to ask fewer rather than more, investigative questions. It is also wise to remember that the *initial* problem which presents is not always the *real* problem, but it takes your skill and enterprise to reach this solution.

You are aware that the time invested in Violet and her twin girls will have a significant impact on the well-being of Violet and the mental and physical development of the twins.

SCENARIO THREE

Raj is a 35-year-old car mechanic who works with his father in their own business. His wife Alia gave birth to a daughter Kimm eight weeks ago. When you visited Alia for her daughter's eight-week check you asked her to complete the EPDS and she had answered 'yes' to the three Whooley questions. This is your third visit.

You have uncovered that Alia misses her mother who lives in another country and finds it difficult to visit her as she is looking after her other daughter who has also recently given birth. Alia is lonely and has few friends as she moved to the town to help with her father-in-law's business but she suffered severe hyperemesis during her pregnancy and has not felt well since. Alia is anxious and finds it difficult to relax. She confides in you that she has been having strange thoughts about her baby, that she feels Kimm seems to be watching her all the time – even when she is out of the room. Sometimes she hears Kimm muttering in a strange voice and thinks she is trying to warn her about something, but she is not sure what. She thinks her daughter is possessed by the Devil. Alia has asked you to keep this confidential as her father-in-law will send her back to her home country as he would think she is mad.

- What are your first impressions?
- What are the possible positive aspects of each impression?
- What are the possible negative aspects of each impression?
- What will you do next?
- How will you proceed?

- **What are your first impressions?**

  Alia sounds as if she is suffering from some hallucinations.

- **What are the possible positive aspects?**

  Alia has felt she can trust me by confiding in me.

- **What are the possible negative aspects?**

  Alia seems to believe that her daughter is possessed.

  Alia might harm her daughter if she feels threatened.

  Alia is not making sense.

- **What are the possible positive aspects?**

  Alia might be encouraged to talk more about her feelings of paranoia and fear.

  I should consider this as a safeguarding issue and keep Alia talking.

- **What are the possible negative aspects?**

  Alia might feel threatened and stop talking if I look alarmed.

  I should consider this as a safeguarding issue and stop Alia talking.

- **What will you do next?**

  I will listen to Alia and suggest she and Kimm come to the general practitioner with me to explain how she feels.

If Alia agrees, inform Social Services about Alia's condition and her ability to care for Kimm.

If Alia is compliant I will listen to her fears, which are obviously worrying her and try to assure her that she is not under any threat and will help look after and hold Kimm.

■ **What are the possible positive aspects?**

As we have already established a rapport, Alia will feel she can trust me.

Both she and the baby will be safe.

■ **What are the possible negative aspects?**

Alia will refuse to come with me and become angry at my suggestions.

Alia will take the baby and attempt to leave the home.

How will you proceed?

Ring the GP to discuss Alia and Kimm.

Ask for an urgent appointment and accompany Alia to see the general practitioner.

Arrange to see Alia at home, if she has not been admitted to a Mother and Baby Unit.

INDEX

Printed in the United States
by Baker & Taylor Publisher Services